Funding
Health Sciences
Research

A Strategy to Restore Balance

Committee on Policies for Allocating
Health Sciences Research Funds

Division of Health Sciences Policy
INSTITUTE OF MEDICINE

Floyd E. Bloom and Mark A. Randolph, editors

NATIONAL ACADEMY PRESS
Washington, D.C.   1990

362.1
In 7

National Academy Press   •   2101 Constitution Avenue, N.W.   •   Washington, D.C. 20418

Major support for the study was provided by the Lucille P. Markey Charitable Trust and The Pew Charitable Trusts. Other support was contributed by the Institute of Medicine, from its own endowment interest income and from other independent sources, including unrestricted donations received from several leading pharmaceutical companies. The project was assisted in initial stages by the National Research Council Fund (NRC), a pool of private, discretionary, nonfederal funds that is used to support a program of Research Council/Institute of Medicine studies of national issues in which science and technology figure significantly.

The NRC Fund consists of contributions from several sources: a consortium of private foundations, including the Carnegie Corporation of New York, the Charles E. Culpeper Foundation, the William and Flora Hewlett Foundation, the John D. and Catherine T. MacArthur Foundation, the Andrew W. Mellon Foundation, the Rockefeller Foundation, and the Alfred P. Sloan Foundation; the Academy Industry Program, which seeks annual contributions from companies that are concerned with the health of U.S. science and technology and with public policy issues with technological content; and the National Academy of Sciences, the National Academy of Engineering, and Institute of Medicine endowments.

Library of Congress Cataloging-in-Publication Data

Institute of Medicine (U.S.). Committee on Policies for Allocating
   Health Sciences Research Funds.
      Funding health sciences research : a strategy to restore balance /
   Committee on Policies for Allocating Health Sciences Research Funds,
   Division of Health Sciences Policy, Institute of Medicine ; Floyd E.
   Bloom and Mark A. Randolph, editors.
         p.   cm.
      Includes bibliographical references.
      Includes index.
      ISBN 0-309-04343-3
      1. Medicine—Research—United States—Finance. 2. Medical
   sciences—Research—United States—Finance. 3. Medical policy—
   United States—Finance. I. Bloom, Floyde E. II. Randolph, Mark A.
   III. Title.
      [DNLM: 1. Health Policy—United States. 2. Research Support—
   organization & administration. 3. Research Support—trends. W
   20.5 I513f]
   R854.U5I57 190
   362.1'072073—dc20
   DNLM/DLC
   for Library of Congress   90-13400
                                                                                    CIP

iii

125178

KENNETH I. SHINE, Dean, School of Medicine, University of California at Los Angeles, Los Angeles, California

P. DENNIS SMITH, Chairman, Department of Biological Sciences, Wayne State University, Detroit, Michigan

Study Staff

Ruth Ellen Bulger, Director, Division of Health Sciences Policy
Alicia K. Dustira, Study Director
Mark A. Randolph, Co-Study Director
Kyung Sook Lee, Research Associate
Claudette K. Baylor-Flemming, Project Secretary
Kimberly A. Kasberg, Project Assistant
Louise M. Gillis, Project Assistant

Foreword

This report represents the efforts of a distinguished committee of university presidents, academic deans, department chairmen, foundation leaders, and university and industry research scientists, who were presented with the difficult task of reviewing the allocation of funding for research in the health sciences and recommending policies to assure balance in support among the components of this research. It contains a valuable analysis of funding and allocation trends in the biomedical fields.

During the two years that they worked, committee members were faced with a rapidly shifting funding environment for health sciences research. When they began in 1988, the National Institutes of Health funded more than 6,000 new and competing R01 grants. By the time they finished the report, this number had dropped to less than 5,000.

At a June 1990 forum on supporting biomedical research sponsored by the National Academy of Sciences (NAS) and the Institute of Medicine (IOM) many scientists and administrators from the public and private sectors expressed serious concerns about the inadequate funds available to support research, especially by young investigators. Both this report and the sense of the forum emphasize that high priority should be given to the training of the next generation of scientists. However, the consensus view of the forum was that we are now facing a crisis in funding of research projects. Thus it may appear incongruous that this report focuses on long-range recommendations calling for more money for training, career development, facilities, and greater flexibility in the calculation of indirect costs. We recognize that in the current environment the committee might also have addressed and highlighted the immediate funding pressures.

It is encouraging that the government officials present at the forum acknowledged the seriousness of the short-term funding problem and announced that they will address the matter in the next budget cycle. It is appropriate therefore that this report seeks to examine long-term strategies that might protect the environment from the wide swings of the past 2 to 3 years and provide long-term stable supplies of investigators, as well as adequate infrastructure to assure the continuing productivity of biomedical research in the country.

This report, like the June Forum, is a manifestation of the continuing concern of the NAS and IOM that adequate funding, properly apportioned, be provided for biomedical research. Our institutions will continue to examine these issues as the research scene and funding patterns change.

FRANK PRESS   SAMUEL O. THIER
President   President
National Academy of Sciences   Institute of Medicine

Preface

Few topics provoke as much intense debate among the participants and policymakers of health sciences research as the processes by which research sponsors decide how much to spend and how to allocate their funds. Almost everyone will acknowledge that health sciences research in the United States has experienced progressive expansion and a remarkable course of accomplishment since Vannevar Bush and his colleagues opened the highway of federally funded discovery at the end of World War II. But, not unlike Mark Twain's comments on the weather, the process of allocating funds for U.S. health sciences research seems to be an issue that draws constant complaints and fuels our desire to do something about it. Important policy decisions on how to expend funds most effectively on research operations, research training, and research equipment and facilities have become issues of intense debate, interminable consternation, and frequent misconceptions both among those providing the funds and those competing to receive them.

From the 1950s through the 1970s, the federal government increased its investment in health sciences research, outstripping the still significant contributions of private foundations that were once the primary sponsors of academic medical science. As other federal programs drew increasingly upon the funds the nation was willing to commit for health research through the 1970s, the rate of federal expansion slowed, but nevertheless retained continuous, albeit modest, growth. A variety of short-term administrative procedures enacted in the 1980s attempted to stretch the available funds to the maximum while simultaneously stabilizing the research base through established minimum numbers of funded research projects and increasing award periods. However, these short-term repairs implemented in a new era of enormous federal budget deficits combined with austere domestic spending policies have, in turn, created new problems. Although the number of projects funded has continued to grow, the number of new grant applications reflecting the awareness of new scientific opportunities has grown even faster. The resulting paradox is that despite the greatest historical federal and private investment in absolute dollars, the probability that any new grant application will be funded has never been lower. This significantly diminished success rate for new research project grant applications is sending painful signals throughout the research ranks.

Along with the growing divergence between the overall health research budget allocation and the increasing proportion of approved but unfunded research projects has come the recognition that important pieces of the health research enterprise have been neglected to keep this gap from growing even wider. Multiple federal and private assessments of the trends in research funding have concluded that we may already be entering a crisis whose effects will not be realized until sometime in the future. Because of the present underattractiveness of health science as a career, the cadre of creative, well-trained health scientists needed to continue our current momentum into the next century is already threatened. Since it takes many years to train medical scientists, these effects will not be realized for several years into the future. The emergence of high-technology biomedical research, and its need for talent to maintain the therapeutic and diagnostic advantages earned by the U.S. health care industry, creates an added but indeterminable need for talent development.

Other surveys have repeatedly documented the degree to which outmoded facilities and equipment have already constrained the potential creativity of the present generation of medical scientists. Yet the problems remain, and the expressions of distress throughout the scientific community grow louder despite the indisputable fact that federal funds and the number of federally funded health research projects are at an all-time high.

In May 1988, the Institute of Medicine appointed the Committee on Policies for Allocating Health Sciences Research Funds to study these potentially onerous trends. It was the committee's task to conduct an in-depth review of the current policies employed by all of the sponsors of health sciences research, including non-federal governmental sources, the private foundations and charitable health agencies, and the corporate health care industry. The committee was also charged to recommend appropriate revisions in these policies in order to restore balance among the essential components of the health research enterprise (research, training, equipment, and facilities); to increase the flexibility in using these funds; and to ensure that, at any established level, the funds committed to health sciences research will be used most effectively to sustain the vitality of the U.S. biomedical research enterprise.

As is customary in studies with such broad implications and potential ramifications, the committee's 18 members were selected to include representation from a broad spectrum of viewpoints including both basic and applied medical researchers; scientific administrators in large and small academic institutions, in private foundations, and in the pharmaceutical industry; and individuals with past direct participation in the administration of federal health sciences research. The breadth of views represented by the committee membership led to intense examination of a large number of perspectives and to the realization that many points of view were in many cases based on inaccurate perceptions of the facts pertaining to amounts contributed by the different sponsors in relation to their research objectives. This report represents the distillation of the factual records on research funding allocations by the various sponsors, and a comprehensive examination of priorities that must be addressed to attain our goal of ensuring the most effective expenditure of the funds to sustain the vigor of our national health research enterprise.

To derive an accurate representation of the current state of funding, the committee received testimony from a large number of research societies, from prominent educators and administrators throughout the health sciences research community, and from a large number of academic scientists and administrators. In addition, three commissioned papers were utilized to bring solid data to bear on the questions of funding trends and gaps in funding, and to illuminate the boundaries of support among the specific sponsors of this research. The committee divided itself into task forces, which, with additional outside participation, focussed on three main sets of issues: the overall strengths and weaknesses of the present system for supporting U.S. health sciences research; the goals of health sciences research; and how to optimize the environment for this research.

Following this assessment of the current trends in research funding, the committee worked toward elaborating a set of objectives for a more idealized research enterprise in which the specific objectives of the sponsors could be more effectively aligned. The most important element in the committee's analysis was developing strategies to attract and retain the most competent and creative scientists. Lastly, the committee worked to develop specific recommendations to re-establish a more balanced research system that begins to redress the consistent underinvestment in some areas of the enterprise. To this end, the committee sought to devise a means to ensure a more balanced and vigorous research enterprise through the participatory interactions of the sponsors, the public, and the scientific community.

The recommendations made are not likely to be seen as the panacea that some would have preferred. In speaking directly to the scientific community, not only about their responsibilities to the system that has spawned them but to their responsibility to the future, we recommend steps to be taken now that may seem in the short term to compromise modestly an already critical period of research project funding. Nevertheless, our intent is to achieve a gradual correction of funding imbalances within the existing system of multiple sponsors. We recommend new processes of policy development, assessment, and continued revision that may reduce the unintended constraints on the system. We propose mechanisms for convening the critical participants, including the scientists, their public supporters, and their critics so that their views of what the future might hold will no longer be captive to the divergent views on how to get there. We also acknowledge that public policy is not static and recommend that the various oversight bodies continuously monitor these and other policy changes that are implemented.

A study of this scope and duration could not have been possible without a dedicated support staff. The committee specifically wishes to acknowledge the solid support provided by the staff of the Institute of Medicine's Health Sciences Policy Division and its director, Ruth Bulger. We recognize the important organizational and administrative contributions made by the original study director, Alicia Dustira, and the writing, analysis, and review steps that were so effectively carried out by her successor, Mark Randolph. Lastly, an especially hearty expression of gratitude is due to Kyung Sook Lee, the research associate, and to Claudette Baylor-Flemming, Kimberly Kasberg, and Louise Gillis for their dedication to our task and their good nature in helping us reach our goals through every known source of communication available to the Institute, from handwritten notes on easel pads to satellite-transmitted telefacsimiles.

> Floyd E. Bloom
> Chairman, Committee on Policies for
> Allocating Health Sciences Research Funds

Contents

Funding
Health Sciences
Research

.

Executive Summary

In the past 40 years the United States has produced the world's preeminent health research enterprise. The success of this enterprise can be attributed both to the generous support of many research sponsors—both public and private—and the use of these funds by health scientists. U.S. scientists have utilized these resources to cultivate a stimulating and creative environment for investigating the fundamental causes of disease in order to improve human health. As a result, health researchers have made great strides in understanding the etiology of such afflictions as cancer, heart disease, diabetes, acquired immune deficiency syndrome (AIDS), mental illness, and drug addiction. These successes have stimulated the continued emergence of an unprecedented array of research opportunities and have challenged scientists to expand the boundaries of knowledge. These opportunities, in turn, have fostered even higher societal expectations of health research and have encouraged researchers to delve deeper into the fundamental causes of disease and their treatment and prevention as well as to increase our understanding of normal biological processes.

Before World War II, industry and private foundations were the primary sponsors of U.S. health-related research. Following the war, however, the amount of government support soon eclipsed that of industry and the private nonprofit sector. The rapid growth in the National Institutes of Health (NIH) (and subsequently the Alcohol, Drug Abuse, and Mental Health Administration [ADAMHA]) reflected the national priority for improving health through fundamental research.

Beginning in the 1970s, however, slower budgetary growth combined

1

with a dramatic inflation rate both reduced the buying power of research dollars and increased the competition for available resources. These forces caused wide fluctuations in the annual number of new and competing grants awarded by the NIH and ADAMHA in the mid to late 1970s. Furthermore, these fluctuations caused uncertainty about the availability of ongoing research support. In response to these concerns, Congress, the NIH, and ADAMHA agreed to stabilize the research base through a policy to fund a fixed minimum number of new and competing research projects each year.

This "stabilization policy" explicitly made individual investigator-initiated research project grants the highest priority for NIH and ADAMHA. Starting with fiscal year 1981, a minimum number of 5,000 new and competing awards was established for NIH; after some compromises between the administration and Congress, 345 were established for ADAMHA. This policy of establishing minimum numbers of new and competing awards was pursued for the following 7 years, during which time new and competing NIH research grants awarded annually grew to all time highs reaching 6,400 by 1987. Similarly, annual grant awards from ADAMHA grew to nearly 600 in the same period.

From 1979 to 1988 the total number of research project grants supported annually by NIH grew by one-third, from 15,500 to nearly 20,900. Similarly, the dollars committed to research project grants grew by 50 percent, from $2.5 billion to $3.9 billion, after adjustments for inflation. The ADAMHA realized similar gains with research grants increasing from 1,250 to more than 1,900, and inflation-adjusted funds growing by 35 percent. These figures seem to indicate that there are now more U.S. scientists engaged in health research with more funds than at any time in the country's history. However, this growth has not been readily acknowledged by many individuals in the scientific community. Additionally, industry is becoming a dominant sponsor in the support of health research and the implication of this trend is presenting challenges to the research environment that were unimagined in the halcyon days of NIH support.

Given this historically unsurpassed level of support, why is there so much concern about the opportunity for adequate research support and the ability to pursue research careers within the biomedical research community? The answers to this question are complex, and based in part, on certain misperceptions of the present status of health sciences research funding.

Although the stabilization policy was important in maintaining a minimum annual number of new and competing awards, the administration's budget requests as well as congressional appropriations for NIH and ADAMHA were never adequate to fund the required number of awards fully. Thus, in order to fund the agreed upon number of new awards, arbitrary administrative cuts, referred to as "downward negotiation," were imposed on the budgets of both competing and continuing research grant awards. This policy may have fostered the perception of federal budget cuts even though the average constant dollar amount of research project grants grew throughout this period. Additionally, in response to other demands from the scientific community, a policy change in the mid-1980s extended the average duration of research grants from 3 to 4 years, and placed additional unfunded commitments on the federal health research budget.

Because of these funding limitations, the number of new and competing grants awarded by NIH dropped from 6,400 in 1987 to 6,200 in 1988, the last year of stabilization. In 1989 the policy for setting the minimum number of grants was halted altogether. Since then the number of new and competing awards has plummeted, dropping to 5,400 in 1989, with an expected decline to 4,600 in 1990. This precipitous decline has sent shockwaves throughout the biomedical community. Simultaneously, the number of grant applications has continued to grow, and the approval rate by peer review panels continues to rise. These trends have further suppressed the proportion of approved grants that were funded from approximately 35 percent in 1988 to less than 25 percent in 1990. Even those scientists fortunate enough to receive project funding have seen downward negotiation cut deeper and deeper into their awards; scientists no longer see a direct relationship among the recommended funding levels approved by the peer review system, the grant awarded by the National Advisory Council, and the amount of funds actually received.

While the policy to stabilize the research base (measured only by the number of competing research projects) initially was effective, it was a short-term solution and did not address the need for longer-term investments. The emphasis on research projects raised speculation that two other vital components of the research infrastructure were being neglected: specifically, training and facilities. As the "baby bust" continues to shrink the labor pool over the next few years, competition for high school graduates in all labor markets will intensify. Moreover, the attrition of scientists trained in the 1950s and 1960s is expected to increase throughout the next decade owing to deaths and retirement. Fewer students and a declining competency in mathematics and science also raise serious concerns about meeting the future demand for well-trained U.S. scientists. At the same time, several comprehensive studies of research facilities and equipment during the 1980s have documented the deteriorating condition of U.S. academic research facilities, and many scientists and science administrators feel that this will hinder their ability to compete successfully for funds to investigate challenging research questions.

Other problems adding pressures to an already strained research establishment have surfaced as well in recent years. These include: (1) an apparent increase in congressional earmarking of funds for research initiatives and facilities construction; (2) large-scale investments to address new national health research priorities (e.g., AIDS, substance abuse, and the Human Genome Project); (3) significantly increased research costs to comply with changes in federal regulations regarding the handling of animals and hazardous waste; (4) federal budgetary constraint imposed by the large federal deficits and deficit reduction legislation; and (5) widespread concern over U.S. economic competitiveness. Thus, a central question facing the nation—and posed by the Institute of Medicine in the charge to this committee—is whether the current resource allocation policies are adequate to sustain our preeminent position?

OBJECTIVES OF THE STUDY

In response to these disturbing trends, the Board of Health Sciences Policy of the IOM proposed a study in which a detailed review of policies for allocating resources for health research would be conducted. For this review a committee of 18 members was appointed that represented the larger community of researchers and administrators in academia, government, industry, and foundations. *The charge to the committee was to analyze the funding sources for research projects, training, facilities, and equipment by federal and nonfederal sources. The committee was asked as well to develop a coordinated set of funding policies to restore balance among these components of the research enterprise in order to ensure optimal use of research dollars for sustaining a vigorous health research enterprise.* The committee was not charged with reviewing the allocation of research support among specific scientific disciplines or disease areas, nor was this policy study intended to be a justification for increasing research funds. Rather, the goal of the study was to ensure that, at any given level of support, allocation policies would enable the scientific community to utilize available resources in the most efficient manner so as to create an optimal research environment and achieve society's goals for research into human disease.

Once established, the committee was divided into task forces that focused on three aspects of the problem: (1) strengths and weaknesses of the current system, (2) goals of health sciences research, and (3) optimization of the health sciences research environment. In addition to drawing on its own expertise, the committee invited written comments and testimony from current and former government officials, congressional staff, foundation and voluntary health agency officials, and administrators in industry and academia. The committee also commissioned background papers to examine the following three issues: (1) overall U.S. funding for biomedical research from both governmental and nongovernmental sources; (2) funding of the research enterprise through NIH and ADAMHA, and (3) the current status of biomedical research facilities.

FINDINGS AND CONCLUSIONS

The committee concluded that the allocation policies of the past decade have focused too heavily on short-term problems and solutions and have neglected the long-term integrity of the research enterprise. The committee reached a consensus that the goals of health research can be achieved only by creating a positive research environment for health sciences. This environment should:

• identify and encourage young talented individuals to pursue health research careers,

• provide stable research support for talented scientists throughout their careers,

• offer flexibility in allocating resources to foster creativity and meet changing demands, and

• provide adequate modern laboratories and equipment necessary for scientific research and training.

These attributes, in turn, will require effective coordination and leadership from the federal research agencies; competent, objective public and private sector administration; and responsiveness to the wishes of the American people through the political process. In the committee's view, the key to future success in the research system is sustained high levels of support for people, projects, and facilities.

The committee analyzed resource allocation policies for each of these components over the past several decades. In terms of capital investment relative to productive life expectancy the committee determined the following:

• The most critical and longest-term investment in the research system is the development of career scientists who contribute to the long-term success of the enterprise through both their own research efforts and their training of future generations of scientists.

• Of a slightly shorter expected lifetime of utility to the enterprise is the capital investment in facilities.

• Finally, individual research projects and equipment generally are the shortest and the most variable investments relative to time.

The committee then ascertained that those elements with the longest survival value (namely the research work force and research facilities) may be resilient enough to withstand temporary budget exigencies in deference to the immediate needs of components with shorter investment periods (research projects and equipment). In practice, emphasis on the short-term needs of the research enterprise has led to underemphasis on funding for the training pipeline and facilities. Therefore, short-term policies favoring support of one component over the others may be acceptable for brief periods, but continuance of such short-term policies may threaten the long-term integrity of the entire system.

To achieve the long-term goals in health sciences research successfully with existing research allocations, the committee believes that attention must be paid to management strategies and policies that look beyond the current crisis in research funding. Thus, the committee's recommendations fall into six general categories that, taken together, can provide for a strong, productive, and self-sustaining health research enterprise. These include the following: (1) a priority-setting framework, (2) a reallocation of existing and future resources to restore appropriate balance among, (3) people, (4) projects, (5) facilities and equipment, and (6) establishing deliberative processes through which sponsors and researchers can communicate and work together to ensure the long-term success of health research. Adoption of these recommendations should provide for an optimum enterprise at whatever level of resources the nation chooses to commit.

RECOMMENDATIONS

Recommendation 1: The committee recommends that Congress, NIH and ADAMHA administrators, and scientists employ a priority-setting framework for allocating funds to meet long- and short-term research needs in order to correct and maintain the appropriate overall balance among the individual components of the research establishment (people, projects, and facilities).

Several interlocking levels of priority setting and decision making must be considered when allocating research funds:

- the total appropriations to all federal agencies receiving funds for health sciences research, including NIH and ADAMHA;
- the allocation within each institute of NIH and ADAMHA for research and training needs;
- the allocations within specific research program areas;
- the allocation of awarded grant funds for a specific research project contributing to the goals of the research program; and
- the total allocation of funds to universities, hospitals, and research institutions that will assume fiscal responsibility for the funds, administer them, and provide the infrastructure for the research projects.

Each program area within each institute or agency has specific needs to address in order to accomplish its mission at any given level of support. However, the desired balance among the components will differ depending on the area of research being supported. Within these established goals, an estimated amount of funds for investigators, research facilities, and research projects (with equipment as a proportion of project funds) will be required over a period of time. Considering that research is made up of a series of such long-term goals, it will be necessary to:

• replenish a certain percentage of talented investigators,
• renovate or replace a certain percentage of buildings or renew equipment, and
• support a certain level of research activity in order to preserve the integrity of the overall system and meet long-term research goals.

The objective of this framework is not to produce one overriding formula that can be applied across the spectrum. Rather, it is to allow for determining priorities among competing needs in the research enterprise. This framework serves as a guideline to mesh broad national health research priorities of individual scientists. The committee emphasizes the importance of designing a priority-setting and resource need assessment process that will allow flexibility in addressing all of the needs of the research enterprise. The committee also emphasizes the need for continuous monitoring of resource allocations to each of the components of the research establishment in order to prevent future imbalances.

REBALANCING HEALTH SCIENCES RESEARCH FUNDS

Recommendation 2: The committee recommends that NIH reallocate its extramural health research funds over the next ten years.

The committee concluded that allocation policies over the past two decades have forced an overall imbalance in the health sciences research system in which support for research project grants has been heavily favored at the expense of training and facilities. Re-establishing balance of funding among research, training, and facilities is crucial for maintaining a vigorous research enterprise and sustaining our international preeminence in health research.

In order to make up for past deficiencies in training allocations throughout the 1980s, and to meet higher personnel demands towards the end of the 1990s, the committee feels that an accelerated growth of the training budget is necessary. The committee emphasizes that there is an integral relationship between research and training. Since an estimated one-quarter of NIH and ADAMHA support for research training is accomplished indirectly through research project grants, allocation policy can not be separated easily into research and training components. However, for defining allocation policy, and in the absence of better data on research project grant funded training, these functions can be treated independently. The committee feels the research community must develop and implement corrective strategies now to avert a work force crisis later in this decade.

To address the funding imbalances, the committee developed allocation strategies under four budget scenarios for balanced funding through the 1990s: (1) no real growth in the health sciences research budget (i.e., no growth beyond inflation); (2) two percent annual real growth; (3) four percent annual real growth; and, (4) possible allocation strategies for budgetary growth higher than four percent.

1. No Real Growth: Even in the event of no average real growth in the health sciences research budget during the 1990s, the committee recommends that funds for training future generations of health scientists be increased incrementally from 4.20 to 5.75 percent of the total extramural research budget by 1995 and to 6.75 percent by the year 2000. Concurrently, the committee recommends that extramural construction funds be increased incrementally from the present 0.25 percent of the extramural budget to 0.50 percent by 1995 and maintain this level through the end of the decade.

This redistribution of funds to training and facilities should come from the increased congressional appropriations, and not reduce the pool of funds for research (Figures 7-1 and 7-2) (Appendix Table A-22). However, in real terms (dollars adjusted for inflation) there will be a slight reduction of research funds under this proposal. This proposal calls for shifting 0.20 percent of the research budget annually (or about $12 million constant dollars per year) to the training budget each year for the next decade. Using an average cost per full-time training position (FTTP) equivalent of $24,000, this proposal would re-allocate enough funds to increase FTTPs by nearly 400 per year. **The committee believes that this growth in the training budget will not enlarge the research project grant applicant pool; rather, the net effect of this gradual reallocation will be to replace the increasing number of scientists expected to retire later this decade.** Furthermore, this recommendation parallels that recommended in the NRC report, *Biomedical and Behavioral Research Scientists: Their Training and Supply.*

The minor shift of funds for extramural construction will merely allow the NIH to meet the most urgent facilities crises. **The committee cannot recommend shifting larger proportions of federal health sciences research funds into the construction category at a time when an increasing number of research grants are not funded fully.** On the other hand, the complete absence of funds authorized for construction could jeopardize the building and renovating of facilities that are crucial to scientific progress.

The committee recommends that a small percentage of funds be restored to the centers and other grants category over the next decade as well. The proportion of extramural funds committed to centers has declined steadily throughout the 1980s. The continued decline in support for centers could diminish the quality of the research conducted in these environments.

It becomes all the more important to increase the support for centers which can serve as technology transfer sites for the translation of research results into clinical practice. Funds transferred to this category could be used for the growing number of interdisciplinary and multi-center disease prevention and epidemiological studies. Also included in this budget category under other grants are funds for the Biomedical Research Support Grant (BRSG) program. Providing more funds through the BRSG program could enhance the abilities of research institutions to assist their young investigators at the local level and may help stabilize the research efforts of mid-career scientists if the traditional grant system becomes even more unpredictable (see recommendation 4.6).

Shifting funds away from research to training and facilities will have some negative ramifications. Over the next decade, the cost of these reallocations will be about $20 million (constant dollars) per year out of an annual $3.8 billion research project grant budget (1988 total). Since these funds would be reallocated from a variety of research programs, the reductions in the traditional (R01) investigator-initiated research project grant pool would be minimized.

2. Two Percent Real Growth: In the event that the health sciences research budget grows, in real terms, an average of two-percent annually, the committee again recommends that funds be reallocated to training and facilities in the same proportions as in the zero growth scenario— training funds increased incrementally from 4.20 to 5.75 percent of the total extramural research budget by 1995 and to 6.75 percent by 2000, and extramural construction funds increased incrementally from the present 0.25 percent of the extramural budget to 0.50 percent by 1995 and through the end of the decade. The real growth in the budget in concert with the reallocations will add more funds to training and facilities budgets without decreasing the research grant budget.

Under this scenario, if the NIH and ADAMHA research budgets grow by two percent annually in real terms (equivalent to the average annual real growth in the NIH budget throughout the 1980s), the committee feels that portions of the net increase also should be shifted to training and facilities (Figures 7-1 and 7-3) (Appendix Table A-23). Throughout the 1980s, no real growth occurred in the training budget category. The small percentage of reallocated funds added to the average annual real growth will reinforce the training commitment of NIH and ADAMHA. While the net growth would allow for increasing the number of FTTPs, the committee feels that some of these augmented training allocations should be used to improve training programs and address insufficient stipend levels (see recommendation 3 below). The percentage of the research budget allocated to facilities will not change from the zero-growth scenario since proportionately more funds will be available due to growth in the overall budget; and, in any case, the amounts needed to reach the estimated facilities construction requirement (see chapter 6) cannot be drawn from the existing sums.

The committee emphasizes that these reallocations will preserve the same or higher level of research effort by not reducing the research portion of the budget in real terms. In fact, if the average size of research project grants remains constant ($184,000 in 1988) through the next decade, the total number of grants supported by NIH could potentially grow from the present level of 20,300 to nearly 24,000. Although the number of funded research grants will grow by about 360-370 per year over the decade, the success rate for applicants will remain relatively unchanged (presently about 24 percent) if the annual number of applications continues to exceed the present 19,500 level.

3. Four Percent Real Growth: In the event that the health sciences research budget grows on an average of four percent annually, the committee recommends that funds for training be incrementally increased from 4.20 percent to approximately 5.4 percent of the total extramural research budget by 1995 and to 6.2 percent by 2000. Reallocating funds for construction should follow the same pattern as the two previous scenarios: incrementally increasing construction funds to 0.50 percent of the extramural budget.

The target percentages for funds to be reallocated to training under the four-percent growth scenario are somewhat smaller than the figures in the two-percent and zero-growth scenarios (Figures 7-4 and 7-5) (Appendix Table A-24). Although the overall percentage of the extramural budget committed to training is less under this scenario, the funding level would actually increase more rapidly due to the growth of the overall budget. Obviously, faster growth of the training budget would eventually outpace the resources available to support the net increase in researchers.

A four percent annual real growth in research funds would allow for a modest expansion of the research base over the next ten years. The net increase in available research funds would allow for the overall number of NIH research project grants to expand gradually, at a rate of about 1000 per year at 1988 grant sizes from the present 20,300 to about 29,400. In 1991 alone, this would raise the annual number of new and competing awards to approximately 6,000. However, with applications exceeding 19,500 and expected to go even higher, the annual success rate will only approach 28 to 30 percent. The committee believes that even at this pace of budget growth a large number of high quality research proposals will go unfunded.

4. More Rapid Growth: The committee also considered the possibility that the NIH and ADAMHA budgets would grow at a more rapid pace, and what the longer term ramifications of such growth might be. The committee was convinced from the data and testimony it received that if all grant parameters (i.e., average grant size and duration, and the annual number of applications) were to remain constant the national health research effort could effectively utilize resources growing at a much higher rate. A larger research effort could build more effectively and rapidly upon the previous accomplishments in health research and further broaden our knowledge of human biology and disease. For example, simply to regain the 35 per cent grant success rate that existed between 1980 and 1987, would require funds for approximately 7000 new and competing awards annually. Using the allocation proportions described above would require an 8 per cent annual real growth.

The overall allocation of funds among extramural research projects, training, and facilities will depend upon the particular needs of the scientists performing research within various scientific programs and disciplines, and the granting mechanisms deployed to meet the goals of these research programs. The committee's suggested allocations are directed towards the overall distribution of funds in order to strengthen the research enterprise by ensuring adequate, but balanced, support to all components of the research enterprise. The committee has not specifically examined the proportion of funds expended on intramural research within any given NIH/ADAMHA institute. This issue has been examined recently by another IOM study group. Growth in the intramural programs is guided by program objectives and advisory councils' oversight, and is constrained by space limitations and employment ceilings.

Within these guidelines, the committee emphasizes that any funds to be redistributed should be drawn first from increases in the annual federal appropriations. However, even in the event of no-real growth in the federal health research budget, the committee firmly endorses that incremental increases in training funds be reallocated from the nominal increases in the overall extramural budget (funds not adjusted for inflation). Under circumstances of real growth, the proposed training increases should come from the new funds so as to detract minimally from the ongoing research effort. Furthermore, the committee emphasizes the importance of making gradual reallocations in order to maintain stability of research support.

The committee is aware that this proposal may be unfavorably received by the scientific community at a time when research grants are not funded fully and research careers appear to be in jeopardy. While these short-term problems abound, the committee is making these recommendations with concern for the long-term integrity of the research enterprise. The earlier IOM report on *Resources for Clinical Investigation* has recommended that 1000 clinical investigation training positions be made available. Additionally, the next biomedical and behavioral manpower report by the NAS to be released in 1992 is expected to review closely the need for increasing the number of physician scientists as well as the doctoral pool. If the federal research budget grows in real terms, and continued monitoring by the NRC Committee on Biomedical and Behavioral Workforce Needs demonstrates an increasing demand for physician scientists, the proposed shift of funds to the training budget would make resources available for implementing these changes. Additionally, adjustments to the research granting system presented below are designed to stabilize research careers through additional steps and to ensure a vigorous, albeit constrained, health research establishment.

TALENT RENEWAL

Recommendation 3: The committee recommends an approach to restore balance in the development of talent through a broad spectrum of incentives and encouragements.

The long-term success of the health research enterprise depends on the continuous development of a cadre of well-trained, creative scientists. Indeed, there are strong indications that the failure to recruit young, talented individuals into the health sciences will significantly hamper our ability to confront future health research challenges. Over the past decade the number of employment opportunities for health scientists in the private sector has grown faster than those in academia. If this trend continues through the 1990s, the demand for scientists could outstrip supply before the end of the century. Other factors affecting the talent pool will be an increasing retirement rate of scientists trained in the 1950s and 1960s as well as a smaller pool of potential candidates resulting from the "baby bust." Therefore, science policymakers must evaluate scientific work force needs for the next twenty to thirty years in order to develop a plan for replenishing the talent pool. The committee's recommendations target several periods of opportunity in the development of an individual's scientific career. The committee emphasizes that training and research are not dichotomous; rather, they are interdependent factors in the research enterprise and are separated here for ease of discussion.

Recommendation 3.1: The committee recommends that programs be supported by the National Science Foundation (NSF) and the other federal agencies, along with the private sector, to introduce undergraduates to career opportunities in health sciences research.

Current levels of training will determine the future capacity of the scientific work force to conduct research and to train the next generation of health scientists. Students interested in the health sciences need to be introduced to research opportunities that encourage them to continue these studies in graduate or medical school, and such programs should include research experience in association with faculty members who can serve as role models and mentors.

Recommendation 3.2: **The committee recommends that programs be developed by the federal government and the private sector that are designed to encourage more women and minorities to pursue careers in the health sciences.**

Of particular concern with regard to undergraduate science enrollment is the underparticipation of women and minority students. Although some students in these categories are sufficiently prepared for a science and engineering education at the start of their college studies, significantly fewer choose these careers than similarly prepared white males. The committee believes that the current system neglects the diversity of individual needs of students in these underrepresented groups. Undergraduate programs specifically designed to encourage women and minority students to pursue their scientific career aspirations could reverse this trend.

Recommendation 3.3: **The committee recommends that NIH and ADAMHA reestablish a competitive predoctoral fellowship program for individuals.**

At the graduate level of training, the current system heavily favors institutional training grants over individual fellowships. However, the committee believes that a combination of mechanisms to support predoctoral students throughout their studies is important. Through reestablishment of this competitive predoctoral award program, students would be supported directly, allowing them more freedom to select the area of investigation they wish to pursue. Most importantly, direct fellowship awards to students would provide a strong signal that the student is an integral and valued member of the health sciences research enterprise, thus enabling more aggressive recruitment of students into postbaccalaureate health sciences education and training.

Recommendation 3.4: **The committee recommends that the number of physician investigators—active and in training—be assessed. Assuming a real decline in the number of physician-scientists, the committee further recommends reallocating resources in order to create a more formal system for training physician-scientists, including curriculum requirements. In addition, experimental federally-funded training programs in clinical research and public health research training programs also should be established.**

Another concern of the committee is the apparent inability to recruit sufficient numbers of physicians into scientific careers, especially clinical investigators and public health careers. The committee believes it is essential to have physician-scientists engaged in both basic and clinical research. The physician-scientist is the critical link between the knowledge uncovered in the laboratory and the translation of that knowledge into clinical practice and population-based programs.

Recruitment of physicians into research careers is hampered severely by the length of time necessary for clinical training as well as by the difficulty of conducting research during this training period. Additionally, the current unfocused structure of many physician research training experiences does not allow for a sufficient introduction of trainees to scientific project design, research methodology, and statistical analysis. Finally, in the posttraining years, the committee believes there is a "triple threat" to academic physicians; they are expected then to be exceptional researchers, exceptional clinicians, and exceptional teachers and mentors. These pressures probably have discouraged many physicians from remaining actively engaged in research, and they will have to be alleviated in order to interest more physicians in research careers.

Recommendation 3.5: The committee recommends that NIH and ADAMHA modify their FIRST award programs to incorporate a formalized assessment of progress by a scientific panel in the third year.

The committee believes that the period between training and becoming an established scientist is the most sensitive period in the career pathway. The committee feels that the recently created First Independent Research Support and Transition (FIRST) Awards are moving in the right programmatic direction for providing our young scientists entry into the competitive traditional grant system (R01). Considering the nature of the FIRST award, the committee does not feel that the progress of these awardees should or could be comparable to that required in the traditional R01 system. However, to ensure that FIRST investigators are being indoctrinated properly into independent scientific investigation and preparing them to compete for R01s, the committee feels that an interim review would improve the program's success. Furthermore, this would provide an opportunity to redirect the young investigator (if necessary) and ensure that the product of this research, in fact, enhances the body of medical knowledge.

IMPROVING THE RESEARCH PROJECT GRANTS SYSTEM

The committee believes that the research project system needs adjustments to preserve the existing pool of talented scientists as well as to provide entry for young scientists. Because of growing obligations from previous years, NIH and ADAMHA increasingly are unable to fund new and competing renewal grant applications. An all-or-none funding policy has demoralized the research community, especially in the current (1990) fiscal year when the number of new and competing awards is so low. Undoubtedly the drop of nearly 1,800 new starts (a 30 percent reduction) since 1987 will interrupt funding to productive scientists. Without effective policy changes, more scientists will fall out of the system, and others understandably will not choose health research careers. Policies that affect research project support should provide the flexibility to respond to rapidly changing needs, but also should provide stable support to research teams.

Recommendation 4.1: The committee recommends that NIH and ADAMHA, as well as other sponsors of research, develop pilot programs to evaluate step-down or rollover funding for selected grant awards.

A pilot program could evaluate the utility and risks of a transitional funding period during grant renewal. Two possibilities for implementing this concept are:

1. Rollover funding: This first transitional scenario would apply to research project grants awarded for periods of 5 or more years. An NIH/ADAMHA review of competing renewal applications would be convened two years before grant termination (e.g., in year 4 of a 5-year grant) and would lead to one of two possible outcomes:

• An accepted application would allow the research project to continue for an additional 5 years. Thus, the renewal award would provide funding for the fifth year plus an additional 4 years, extending the project to 9 years.

• An unsuccessful competing renewal in year 4 would require that the investigator submit an amended competing renewal application in year 5. If the amended application is then approved, funding would be continued for years 6 through 10.

2. Step-down funding: Another possible transitional funding mechanism would extend partial funding for an additional year for those excellent renewal applications that fail to merit adequately high percentile rankings, and for which revised renewal applications would be invited by the review committee. In such cases the extension year would be funded at a fixed level, such as 60 percent of the last fully funded award period. This type of program would allow investigators to retain key research staff and perform crucial portions of their ongoing research while a revised grant application was being considered.

These are examples of mechanisms that would allow investigators to participate in two consecutive review cycles prior to losing funding.

Recommendation 4.2: The committee recommends that NIH and ADAMHA consider modifying the traditional investigator-initiated grant system (R01) to fund grants on a sliding scale based on percentile ranking.

The compression of grant applications receiving high-priority scores and the necessity of determining a single pay line for funding does not necessarily take into consideration the benefits or potential breakthroughs that could be derived from those grant applications falling below arbitrary cut-offs. The committee believes that the scientific community has to cast a wider net in order to capitalize on excellent opportunities that may fall below the funding cut-off. A sliding-scale funding mechanism could reinforce and protect the best research projects and reduce the suffering from downward negotiation throughout the system. It also would increase the opportunity to sponsor high quality research proposals that are increasingly falling just below an arbitrarily established pay line.

One suggested plan would scale down the award duration or funding level based on such a criterion as the *percentile* ranking. This proposal would encourage investigators to set priorities in their own programs according to their funding level, since those with lower percentages of funding would have to choose which aspects of their research to pursue. This would preserve scientific talent by not forcing investigators out of the system as in the case of a fund/no fund decision. Furthermore, according to the committee's calculations, this strategy would also increase the opportunity for young investigators with novel ideas to gain initial access to the grant system despite inexperience in grant writing.

Recommendation 4.3: The committee recommends that NIH and ADAMHA consider revamping the Small Grants program (R03) for funding innovative, high-risk ideas.

As funds have become more constrained, the committee believes that study sections and institutes have become even more disinclined to fund high-risk research proposals. The committee suggests that NIH and ADAMHA adopt the model of NSF's pilot program called Expedited Awards for Novel Research. The committee emphasizes that this system should not be viewed as an alternative to the peer-review system, but rather should be used as an opportunity to support exciting but high-risk research that would otherwise go unfunded.

Changes in Research Management

Recommendation 4.4: The committee endorses the recommendation by the IOM group studying the NIH Intramural Research Program that Congress annually appropriate to the director of NIH a discretionary fund of no less than $25 million. A discretionary fund also should be appropriated for the ADAMHA administrator. (The committee acknowledges that this proposal is included in the President's 1991 budget.)

The committee concluded that the dynamic nature of the health research environment frequently requires that monies be available to address emerging problems and/or research needs. The committee found that the directors of NIH and ADAMHA are in a unique position to determine specific areas that require urgent attention and that cannot necessarily wait until the next congressional appropriations cycle. An approach to improve flexibility would provide the directors with the resources to initiate activities across institute lines—without intruding on the independence of the individual institutes.

Recommendation 4.5: The committee recommends that the Federal Demonstration Project be expanded as additional experience becomes available.

The Florida Demonstration Project (FDP) was intended to reduce the administrative burden on grantees by streamlining procedures and reducing costs in the federally sponsored project system. Initial reactions to the FDP generally were quite favorable. In October 1988 the project was redesignated the Federal Demonstration Project and was expanded to include 26 institutions. This creative approach is likely to continue to be extremely valuable, for it allows scientists to concentrate more on research than on administrative details.

Recommendation 4.6: The committee recommends that NIH continue to fund the Biomedical Research Support Grant (BRSG) program to universities and research institutions in order to continue flexible program development under institutional control. Furthermore, the committee suggests that the universities and research institutions disburse BRSG funds through faculty peer review groups to support new research initiatives, especially those of young investigators.

The ability of university research administrators to reward young talent and preserve ongoing projects would increase the sense of security among researchers. The committee believes that the BRSG program sponsored by NIH and ADAMHA provides flexibility to university faculty and administrators to support new and ongoing initiatives within their own institutions. The committee believes that the BRSG program has played a significant role in funding young scientists and other institutional initiatives crucial to their overall research and training programs. However, the BRSG program has been a continual target for budget cuts and was slated for elimination by OMB in the early 1980s. Between fiscal years 1989 and 1990, the BRSG program suffered a cut of $11 million, its budget declining from $55.2 to $44.4 million, and it is the target of further reductions in the proposed 1991 budget to $17.7 million. The committee feels that this small commitment to flexibility and researcher security is crucial for initiating and promoting stability in the careers of health scientists.

THE PHYSICAL INFRASTRUCTURE

Correction of inadequate facilities and equipment will have to be gradual, for commitment of a substantial portion of existing federal funding to facilities at this time would create another imbalance in the support for people and projects. Many creative solutions will be necessary to modernize the physical research infrastructure. The most direct approach to the infrastructure crisis is to increase federal funding for health sciences research facilities and equipment. Many believe that renewed federal support for construction and renovation is necessary and that such a program would help stem the flow of direct appeals by individual institutions to Congress for pork barrel appropriations for specific facility development.

Recommendation 5.1: The committee recommends that Congress authorize and appropriate funds for a competitive matching fund construction program to renovate or construct health sciences research facilities, bearing in mind the increased costs of updating facilities to meet recently enacted regulations.

Federal construction programs should focus on renovating existing space as well as funding new construction. Initially, a program could be established without additional appropriations by creating a scientific construction authority and appropriating a portion of the nearly $300 million now being funnelled by Congress to certain institutions through ad hoc pork barrel amendments. These monies would be subject to a comprehensive merit review, taking into consideration both scientific criteria and appropriate socioeconomic and political criteria. The committee feels strongly that pork barreling does not serve the best interests of the nation in the long run and thus should be avoided.

Recommendation 5.2: To allow greater flexibility for institutions to address their own facilities needs, the committee recommends that the sponsors of health research modify indirect cost calculations in the following ways:

1.   The federal government should change federal grant accounting procedures to allow negotiation of separate line items in the IDC recovery rate for facilities renovation and construction separate from that of administrative and library costs.

2.   The federal government should increase IDC use allowance to reduce amortization periods for buildings and equipment.

3. Private foundations, voluntary health organizations, and corporations should observe more closely the true costs of the research they sponsor, including the IDC portion.

Most research buildings become obsolete in 20 years, and equipment often is obsolete 4 to 7 years after purchase. The committee feels that sponsors of health research should link support for particular facilities with individual research projects to allow faster recovery of institutional funds used to maintain facilities and to repay loans used for construction or renovation. In order to accomplish this, research institutions need to have options available to recoup previous expenditures for renewing their research physical plant. This could be done by changing the annual IDC allowance for building amortization from the present 2 percent to 5 percent and by raising the allowance for equipment amortization from 6 2/3 to 20 percent. This would allow research institutions to depreciate their buildings over 20 years rather than 50, and equipment in 5 years rather than 15.

The committee emphasizes that this policy change must not reduce the pool of funds available for direct research costs. The committee links this suggested policy change to one that research institutions limit their IDC rates to current levels, and that they sequester the reimbursed facilities and equipment funds in accounts that will ensure rehabilitation or construction of research buildings and replacement of equipment. Furthermore, this policy change could allow research institutions the flexibility to set their own priorities within their budgets for IDC recovery. Thus, these changes within individual institutional IDC rates will not drive up the overall indirect costs of research reimbursed by the NIH and ADAMHA. The merits of this policy change should be weighed carefully against the unpleasant alternatives of crumbling buildings and inoperable equipment. Inaction now will only exacerbate the growing infrastructure problems at colleges and universities.

Recommendation 5.3: The committee recommends that rules be adjusted so that indirect costs can be applied to direct rental costs of leased facilities.

In some cases research institutions may wish to lease land to a developer who will construct a research facility. The developer may, in turn, lease the space in the research building back to the research institution. In such cases maximum flexibility should be provided so that the building can be leased or purchased through direct or indirect costs associated with research conducted in the facility. Developer interest in these types of projects may be predicated upon tax accounting rules, which may require some accommodation with regard to how rental or overhead funding is provided.

ESTABLISHING AN ONGOING PROCESS FOR RESEARCH PROGRAM MANAGEMENT AND OVERSIGHT

The committee concluded that the present system is becoming increasingly stressed by short-term corrective actions whose long-term consequences have not been fully assessed. Growing federal deficits, earmarking of funds to meet specific health needs, and rigid allocation policies within the health sciences establishment have reduced flexibility within the system. These problems emphasize the need to review federal priorities and coordinate federal health sciences research efforts. Integrating scientific priorities, as determined by peer review or other review mechanisms, with sound policy will lead to more effective resource allocation to improve the overall environment of health sciences research. *While the committee endorses an open forum for discussing priorities and manners of addressing the problems facing health research, it also emphasizes that top-down research directives will be counterproductive to research.*

Failure to maintain constructive policies that integrate the efforts of government and private and nonprofit sponsors of research will limit scientific progress, jeopardize our continued leadership, and imperil our economic strength. It is imperative that review and oversight of the balance among the research components be conducted on an ongoing basis. Therefore, the committee focused on developing mechanisms whereby the sponsors of health sciences research could work cooperatively to monitor progress, develop solutions, and make recommendations to address the problems facing health research. The objectives of this process are

- to optimize the use of resources from all sponsors of health sciences research;
- to improve the nation's capacity to respond to health crises and capitalize on new research opportunities; and
- to restore balance in the components of the system and resource allocation between support for people, projects, and facilities.

Improving Communication Among Federal Agencies

Recommendation 6.1: The committee recommends that a Federal Coordinating Council for Science, Engineering, and Technology (FCCSET) Subcommittee for Health Sciences be established in the Office of Science and Technology Policy (OSTP) to review federal priorities and coordinate federal health sciences research efforts on a continuing basis.

Because of the impact that health-related decisions have on the public, the committee believes it is essential to continue having high level health sciences research advice available to the President through the Office of Science and Technology Policy (OSTP). The committee believes that effective mechanisms are necessary for developing cross-cutting health science policy among the federal scientific agencies, such as the Federal Coordinating Council for Science, Engineering and Technology. The committee believes that advice obtained through the FCCSET Subcommittee on Health will improve intergovernmental communication and cooperation for defining national health sciences research priorities. Ultimately, this will lead to more effective policies for allocating resources for project support, training, and facilities and equipment. While the committee believes that the health sciences FCCSET will address interagency coordination of research, the White House also needs a formal mechanism for obtaining broad scientific advice from nongovernmental scientists. The current director of the OSTP has established a President's Council of Advisors on Science and Technology (PCAST), composed of nongovernmental science experts. *This is the kind of advisory body that the committee envisioned as a means to provide the President and FCCSET with advice from nonfederal scientists.*

Improving Communication Between Federal and Nonfederal Health Sciences Research Sponsors

Recommendation 6.2: The committee recommends that a forum like the Government-University-Industry Research Roundtable (GUIRR) of the National Academy of Sciences be established to review the support of health sciences research on an ongoing basis and to facilitate communication among the various sectors that support health sciences research.

The vitality of the health sciences research enterprise depends not only on federal government activities but the cooperation of all parties involved in health sciences research: universities, independent research institutions, and the private sector (foundations, voluntary health organizations, and corporations). Each must recognize the interdependence of the various sponsors of health science research to maximize its own contributions. These various participants should have a mechanism for open dialogue to facilitate the efficient use of the limited health sciences research resources.

The GUIRR was established by the National Academy of Sciences, National Academy of Engineering, and the IOM to address cross-cutting issues that affect all areas of science and technology. It is composed of scientists, engineers, administrators, and policymakers from all sectors and has as its objective to understand issues, to inject imaginative thought into the system, and provide a setting for discussing and seeking of common ground.

To ensure that the balance of support among components of health sciences research is reestablished and maintained, this review would include evaluation of the relationships among support for research projects, the number of researchers being trained compared to the nation's needs and scientific opportunities, and the status of research facilities. This GUIRR-type committee should include representation from the executive and legislative branches of the federal government, pharmaceutical and biotechnology industries, state governments, academic research institutions, private foundations, and voluntary health agencies. The committee recommends that the proposed committee initially identify the special responsibilities, interests, and contributions of each of these support sources and explore means to achieve health sciences research goals through greater interaction of the sponsors and performers of research.

Recommendation 6.3: The committee recommends that sponsors and researchers explore ways to share facilities and equipment among research institutions, industry, and government.

As equipment and facilities costs continue to soar, cooperative sharing should reduce the need to duplicate investment in physical infrastructure. Even if it cannot be done on a widespread basis, limited cooperation can further advances in health research and possibly reduce unnecessary duplication of capital investments. While conflict of interest must be carefully avoided, the committee is convinced that cooperative agreements can be facilitated without compromising the integrity of researchers or research institutions.

Recommendation 6.4: The committee recommends that foundations and voluntary health organizations maintain their support for new lines of investigation and research projects that, for political or structural reasons, NIH and ADAMHA cannot fund.

Traditionally, foundations and voluntary health agencies have been key supporters of interdisciplinary or innovative projects, or those that for political or other reasons are difficult to support with federal funds. These organizations can respond to new lines of inquiry faster than the government bureaucracy allows. Furthermore, the disease-specific nature of voluntary health agencies provides them with greater focus for supporting innovative ideas in specific areas of investigation as well as funding trainees.

Although the committee believes that foundations and voluntary health agencies are integral to the health research enterprise, it emphasizes that these organizations can not be considered substitutes for federal support. Rather, these organizations should supplement federal efforts and fill in gaps in support in very specific areas of research. Hopefully, by opening more effective lines of communication as described in recommendations 6.1 and 6.2, a more efficient use of scarce resources will be facilitated.

SCIENTIST RESPONSIBILITIES

Federal health research allocation policies often have emerged piecemeal out of the continuing political process. Policy decisions largely reflect scientific, political, and economic influences. The sponsors of health research need to work toward common goals with the research community in order to provide an optimum environment for health research. The committee's recommendations to now have focused primarily on the responsibilities of the sponsors. Little has been said about the role of research scientists and their responsibilities to the research system. Indeed, the key to a viable system is the active participation of scientists in all aspects of the research enterprise, including priority setting and allocation policy.

The committee concluded that research scientists could take actions that would help to improve the future success of the enterprise beyond their own commitment to specific research projects. Scientists should assume a more active role in the policy decision-making process and should champion the overall needs of the research establishment. Health research is a long-term investment, and scientists need to express their views to governmental representatives so that Congress and the Executive Branch can set national research priorities. Scientists also have a responsibility to serve on peer review panels; to review journal articles; and to provide advice on policy boards of the federal government, private foundations, and charitable organizations.

The committee believes that scientists should become more involved in improving the public's understanding of science. Negative publicity about science and scientists seems to be uppermost in the public consciousness in recent years. A small number of highly publicized cases of alleged scientific misconduct and fraud is cited by some to be the tip of an iceberg of deception and misconduct pervading the scientific community. On the other hand, members of the scientific community have argued that the high degree of methodological reproducibility establishes the sound basis of scientific observation. Researchers must continue to show high regard for animal welfare and the proper handling of toxic wastes in order avoid any negative ramifications on the research establishment. To improve the public's opinion of science, the committee believes that scientists must strive to rid the system of misconduct; they must cooperate fully with their institutions and research sponsors in cases of suspected wrongdoing. Also, scientists need to help prevent overreaction to these unfortunate incidents that could easily stigmatize the field. The committee endorses the recommendations of a recent IOM study group report, *The Responsible Conduct of Research in the Health Sciences.* These include recommendations that scientists, individually as well as through professional societies and other organizations, promote high ethical standards in the conduct of research.

Failing to address these concerns in the rapidly paced and highly competitive realm of modern biomedical research could have serious consequences, for each new case of scientific misconduct increases the possibility of federal regulation. The committee is concerned that legislatively mandated guidelines for ethical conduct and scientific reporting could impede research activities and increase research costs.

A CALL TO ACTION

Many of the problems, issues, and opportunities considered by this committee have been tackled before by the scientific community and by advisors to and within government. Despite numerous recommendations by these various groups, no decision to act has been made, and the basic problems therefore have persisted. The present analysis has sought to include all the sources of health sciences research support in order to provide a more comprehensive overview of current trends for all components of the research establishment. The committee concluded that an imbalance in support among the components of the research enterprise needs to be addressed immediately to ensure a viable system into the next century. Effective and longer-term corrections will be made only when those who are examining the issues have the authority to act on their conclusions as well. Therefore, the committee believes that in order to begin to resolve the problems discussed in this report and to make the best use of available research funds, ongoing communication among all research sponsors and the whole of the scientific community is vitally important. Only in this way can the wisdom invested in the enterprise be applied in a continuing effort of self-regulation and success.

1

Introduction

Before World War II health research was supported and conducted predominantly by corporations and private foundations. The federal government played a relatively small role in health research, conducting research primarily in its own laboratories at the National Institutes of Health (NIH). Capitalizing on the contributions of basic research to the war effort, federal science programs expanded rapidly after the war. The prescient words of Vannevar Bush 45 years ago helped establish a policy for government investment in science. Bush recognized both the need for governmental support of basic research in academic settings and the need for federally supported science training programs. He proposed five basic principles that should underlie governmental support of scientific research and education:

1. Whatever the extent of support may be, there must be stability of funds over a period of years so that long range programs may be undertaken.
2. The agency to administer such funds should be composed of citizens selected only on the basis of their interest in and capacity to promote the work of the agency. They should be persons of broad interest in and understanding of the peculiarities of scientific research and education.
3. The agency should promote research through contracts or grants to organizations outside the Federal Government. It should not operate any laboratories of its own.
4. Support of basic research in the public and private colleges, universities, and research institutes must leave the internal control of policy,

25

personnel, and the method and scope of the research to the institutions themselves. This is of the utmost importance.

5. While assuring complete independence and freedom for the nature, scope, and methodology of research carried on in the institutions receiving public funds, and while retaining discretion in the allocation of funds among such institutions, the Foundation proposed herein must be responsible to the President and the Congress. Only through such responsibility can we maintain the proper relationship between science and other aspects of a democratic system.[1]

Although these principles initially were proposed for establishing the National Science Foundation (NSF), they were adopted readily by the health research community. Increasing appropriations and flexible research policies enabled the NIH to expand its research programs beyond the federal laboratories through a variety of extramural programs. Throughout the 1950s and 1960s, in what may be referred to as the "golden era" of health research, the federal government provided generous funding for research and training as well as support for building modern research facilities. The growing level of investment during this period resulted in tremendous scientific and clinical advances. Indeed, in this time the United States produced the world's preeminent health research enterprise.

Beginning in the 1970s, however, slower budgetary growth combined with a dramatic inflation rate both reduced the buying power of research dollars and increased the competition for available resources, which then prompted wide fluctuations in the annual number of new and competing grants awarded by NIH and the Alcohol, Drug Abuse, and Mental Health Administration (ADAMHA). Furthermore, these fluctuations caused uncertainty about the availability of ongoing research support. In response to these concerns, Congress, the NIH, and ADAMHA agreed to stabilize the research base through a policy to fund a fixed minimum number of new and competing research projects each year. This "stabilization policy" explicitly made individual investigator-initiated research project grants the highest priority for NIH and ADAMHA.

In fiscal year 1981 a minimum number of 5,000 new and competing awards was established for NIH. Initially, a minimum number of 570 awards was proposed for ADAMHA, but the administration's budget request for 1981 cut the number to 284; Congress then increased the target to 345. This policy of establishing minimum numbers of new and competing awards was pursued for the following 7 years. Over this period new and competing awards from NIH grew to all time highs, reaching 6,400 in 1987. Likewise, over the same period new and competing awards grew to nearly 600 for ADAMHA.

From 1977 to 1988 the total number of research project grants supported by NIH grew by one-third, from 15,500 to nearly 20,900. Similarly, the dollars committed to research project grants grew by 50 percent, from $2.5 billion to $3.9 billion, after adjustments for inflation. The ADAMHA realized similar gains. Thus, it appears there are now more U.S. scientists engaged in health research with more funds than at any time in the country's history.

Given this historically unsurpassed level of support, why is there so much distress and concern about the opportunity for adequate research support and the pursuit of research careers within the biomedical research community? The answers to this question are complex and based, in part, on certain misperceptions of the present status of health sciences research funding.

Although the stabilization policy was important in maintaining a minimum annual number of new and competing awards, the administration's budget requests, as well as congressional appropriations for NIH and ADAMHA never were adequate to fund the required number of awards fully. This has led to arbitrary administrative cuts, referred to as "downward negotiation," in the budgets of both competing and continuing research grant awards in order to fund the agreed-upon number of new awards. Despite this downward negotiation, however, the average dollar amount of research project grants grew throughout this period. Additionally, a policy change to extend the duration of research grants was instituted in the mid 1980s, which has increased the average length of grant awards from 3 to 4 years.

The number of new and competing awards by NIH dropped from 6,400 in 1987 to 6,200 in 1988, the last year of stabilization, and in 1989 the policy for setting the minimum number of grants was halted altogether. Since then, the number of new and competing awards has plummeted, dropping to 5,400 in 1989, and it is expected to decrease to 4,600 in 1990—a decline that has sent shock waves throughout the biomedical community. Simultaneously, the number of grant applications and their approval rate by peer review panels continue to rise, a trend that further suppresses the award rate which has fallen from 35 percent to less than 25 percent in the past 2 years. Even those fortunate enough to receive project funding have seen downward negotiation cut deeper and deeper into their awards. Scientists therefore no longer see a direct relationship among the amount of funding recommended by the study section, the amount awarded by the national advisory councils, and the amount of funds actually received.

Although this policy to stabilize the research base was effective, it was a short-term solution, and therefore did not address the need for longer-term investments. The emphasis on numbers of research projects fueled concern that other vital components of the research infrastructure were being neglected—specifically training and facilities. By many estimates, the supply of scientists will be grossly inadequate to meet future demands. Indeed, between 1972 and 1989 research training as a percent of research and development (R&D) grants in NIH dropped steadily from 15 percent to nearly 4.3 percent. Moreover, attrition of scientists trained in the 1950s and 1960s is expected to increase through the next decade from deaths and retirement, and as the "baby bust" continues to shrink the labor pool over the next few years, competition for high school graduates in all labor markets will intensify. Additionally, fewer students and a declining student competency in mathematics and science raise serious concerns as well about meeting the future demand for well-trained U.S. scientists.

Of no less concern is the condition of U.S. research facilities and equipment. Several comprehensive studies of research facilities and equipment during the 1980s documented the deteriorating condition of our academic research infrastructure. Federal investment in health research facilities has declined precipitously since 1970. Only three NIH institutes (the National Cancer Institute, the National Heart, Lung and Blood Institute, and the National Eye Institute) now have construction authority, and appropriations for these throughout the 1980s were negligible. Many scientists and science administrators feel that the deteriorating condition of facilities and equipment will hinder their ability to successfully compete for the funds necessary to investigate challenging research questions.

Other problems have surfaced in recent years that put added pressures on an already strained research establishment. Many scientists believe that Congress has assumed the responsibility for making important scientific decisions. This is reflected through an increasing practice of earmarking funds for research initiatives and facilities construction in legislation. Large-scale investments to address national priorities, such as AIDS, substance abuse, and the Human Genome Project, are increasing competition for already-scarce research resources. Additionally, changes in federal regulations concerning the handling of animals and hazardous waste, although decidedly important, are costly and will consume increasing amounts of research dollars.

At a time of great scientific opportunity, our nation's ability to invest in health sciences research is being limited by large federal deficits, and although appropriations for NIH and ADAMHA have been growing slowly over the past decade, they are subject to the same fiscal constraints as other federal programs during this time of federal deficit reduction. At the same time, global competitiveness has heightened as the coalescence of the European Economic Community approaches in 1992 and political changes reshape Eastern Europe. A new biotechnology industry making pioneering advances in diagnostics, vaccines, and novel medications is emerging as a formidable arena of international competition. Success in this arena hinges not only on research discoveries but also on our ability to apply knowledge gained. Thus, the United States must maintain its momentum in health research while contending with the need to reduce the federal deficit. A central question facing the nation—and posed by the Institute of Medicine in the formation of this committee—is whether the current resource allocation policies are adequate to sustain the United States preeminent position or whether these policies will lead to a steady erosion of U.S. R&D in the health sciences.

OBJECTIVES OF THE STUDY

In response to the disturbing trends discussed above, the Board of Health Sciences Policy of the IOM proposed a study to conduct a detailed review of policies for allocating health research resources. For this review a committee of 18 members was appointed that represented the larger community of researchers and administrators in academia, government, industry, and foundations. The committee was asked both to analyze the funding sources for research projects, training, facilities, and equipment by federal and nonfederal sources, and then to develop a coordinated set of funding policies to restore balance among these components of the research enterprise in order to ensure optimal use of research dollars for sustaining a vigorous health research enterprise. The committee was not asked to review the allocation of research support among specific scientific disciplines or disease areas, nor was the policy study intended to be a justification for increasing research funds. Rather, the goal of this study was to ensure that, at any given level of support, allocation policies would enable the scientific community to utilize available resources in the most efficient manner in order to create an optimal research environment and achieve society's goals for research into human disease.

The committee was divided into task forces focusing on three aspects of the problem: (1) strengths and weaknesses of the current system, (2) the goals of health sciences research, and (3) optimization of the environment for health sciences research (Appendix C). In addition to drawing on its own expertise, the committee invited written comments and testimony from current and former government officials, congressional staff, foundation and voluntary health agency officials, and administrators in industry and academia (Appendix D). The committee also commissioned the following three background papers:

1. "U.S. Funding for Biomedical Research, An Update of the 1985 Report Prepared for the Pew Charitable Trusts," by Z. E. Boniface.

2. "Organizational Structure and Funding Trends of NIH and ADAMHA," by M. A. Randolph.

3. "The Current Status and Perceived Needs of Biomedical Research Equipment and Facilities," by D. K. Abbass.

BOUNDARIES AND GOALS OF HEALTH SCIENCES RESEARCH

To identify the scientific fields relevant to this study, the committee found it necessary to define the boundaries of health research. To this end, the committee adopted the range of disciplines presented in a 1979 IOM report—*DHEW's Research Planning Principles: A Review.*[2] This range follows a continuum from basic discovery to applied health care and is summarized here:

- the biomedical sciences, which inquire into the basic nature of life through deeper understanding of life processes;
- the clinical sciences, which translate fundamental research into medical practice;
- the population-based sciences, such as epidemiology and biostatistics;
- the behavioral and social sciences;
- biophysics, bioengineering, and clinically oriented medical engineering and physics;
- the hybrid sciences, such as nutritional and environmental sciences;
- health services research, which studies the health care system; and
- technology transfer.

Additionally, the committee members worked from the premise that there is too little emphasis on research into disease prevention as well as in the emerging field of outcomes research (which compares the effectiveness of various treatments and/or therapies). And that therefore the following goals must be considered when developing any new policies to allocate research funds:

- advancing the fundamental knowledge base of the health sciences;
- translating fundamental knowledge into improved diagnostic, treatment, and preventive interventions and thereby helping to alleviate suffering, improve the quality of life, and enhance survival;
- providing the basis for regulatory actions designed to promote safety and health; and
- providing the basis for informed decision making on health policy matters, including the organization, delivery, and financing of health care.

Within the context of these goals, the committee's primary task was to develop a framework for policy decisions promoting successful research in an environment that identifies, encourages, and promotes creativity. Such an environment must provide stable support for talented scientists, flexibility and appropriate allocation of resources to meet changing demands, and laboratories and equipment that meet the scientist's needs. When the research environment is positive, supportive, and reasonably optimistic, it encourages the recruitment of new investigators and fosters the creativity of talented health researchers.

This report thus focuses on the *process* of supporting the health sciences research enterprise, the *people* involved in the research, the *project support system* itself, and the need to restore *facilities and equipment*. In this regard, all of the committee's recommendations were designed for a threefold purpose. First, scientists should be educated and trained adequately for whatever branch of health sciences research they find stimulating. Second, adequate and varied grant mechanisms should be available for researchers to follow creative and meritorious endeavors throughout their scientific careers. Third, laboratories must have adequate space and sufficient modern equipment for U.S. health scientists to continue performing world-class research and to train the next generation of health scientists. The optimal research environment is not a minimum (or maximum) number of partially funded grants but is instead a stable but flexible research environment.

The committee traced the development of the U.S. system for supporting research and reviewed current policies for allocating research funds. In light of the magnitude of the current U.S. investment in health sciences research, as well as recent economic, demographic, and political developments that affect funding and administration of research programs, the committee felt that better mechanisms for long-range planning and coordination of research support could improve the use of research dollars. Definition of this coordination takes two forms: (1) coordinating support for health sciences research within the federal establishment and (2) simultaneously, increasing communication among federal and non-federal sponsors of research. The primary objective of the recommendations in this report is to focus on the need for a forum for both communicating among supporters of health sciences research and encouraging them to develop long-range plans. It is vitally important that these processes be part of a continuous effort to monitor and revise policies to ensure the continued vigor in the nation's health sciences research enterprise.

REFERENCES

1. Bush, V. 1945. Science—The Endless Frontier, A Report to the President on a Program for Postwar Scientific Research. Washington, D.C.: Office of Scientific Research and Development. (Reprinted by the National Science Foundation, May 1980.)
2. Institute of Medicine. 1979. DHEW's Research Planning Principles: A Review. Washington, D.C.: National Academy Press.

2

Funding for Health Sciences Research

The United States is widely recognized as the world's greatest investor in health sciences research. Of the estimated $132 billion invested in all research and development (R&D) in the United States in 1989, $20.6 billion was health related (Figure 2-1).[1,2] In this country health research is funded by three autonomous yet interlocking sectors: (1) federal, state, and local governments; (2) industry; and (3) private nonprofit organizations. In 1988 the federal, state, and local governments supported slightly more than half (51 percent) of all health-related R&D in the United States. Of the remainder, industry supported about 45 percent, and private nonprofit organizations supported about 4 to 5 percent (Figure 2-1). This ratio has changed slightly over the past decade, while the nation's investment in health research has tripled in current dollars (Figure 2-2). In inflation-adjusted dollars the investment has grown by 65 percent during this time (Figure 2-3).

Before World War II, however, the federal government did not invest heavily in life sciences R&D. Most federal support for biological research was sponsored by the Department of Agriculture through block grants to the land-grant colleges. Projects sponsored by these funds were targeted toward the applied life sciences of agriculture and forestry, with few provisions for basic biological research. Additionally, geographical criteria were employed as the primary means to disburse these funds.

During this same period, health research was sponsored primarily by industry, academic institutions, and private individuals.[3] In fact, of the

32

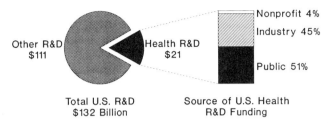

Total U.S. R&D
$132 Billion

Source of U.S. Health
R&D Funding

FIGURE 2-1 Estimated U.S. research and development expenditures for 1989.[1,2]

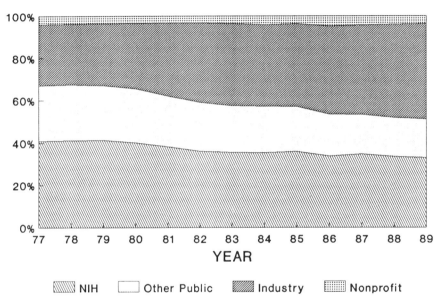

NIH ☐ Other Public ▨ Industry ▦ Nonprofit

FIGURE 2-2 Source of U.S. support for health research and development from 1977 to 1989.[2]

estimated $45 million spent on biomedical research in 1940, industry contributed 55 percent or about $25 million. Approximately 26 percent ($17 million) came from philanthropy, either through earnings on institutional endowments or grants from foundations. The federal government's investment that year totaled $3 million—about 15 percent of the total, most of which was spent in its own laboratories. Some university-based investigators eschewed governmental support, fearing the loss of intellectual freedom and undue influence on their research.[4]

During World War II, basic research in the sciences made significant contributions to the success of the war effort. In 1945 Vannevar Bush, then

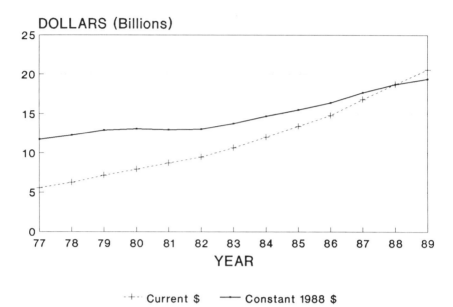

DOLLARS (Billions)

YEAR

·-+-· Current $ ——— Constant 1988 $

FIGURE 2-3   Total U.S. support for health research and development from 1977 to 1989. (Appendix Table A-1)

head of the Office of Scientific Research and Development (OSRD), formulated a set of proposals intended to sustain the nation's war-time research momentum and direct it toward civilian goals. His report to the President, entitled "Science, the Endless Frontier," proposed a coordinated federal policy of investing in research and training new researchers.[5] The policy was to be driven by scientific merit rather than by political or geographical interest. Subsequently, Bush and his colleagues in OSRD established a system by which grants and contracts were awarded to institutions based on scientific merit, and this approach became the cornerstone of the peer-reviewed, academically based system now in place for federally sponsored, competitive extramural research grant programs.

In the two decades following the war, several pieces of legislation changed the organization and conduct of scientific research in the United States. The federal government became the largest single sponsor of health research and about three fifths of these funds now come from programs in the Department of Health and Human Services (DHHS), namely those in the Public Health Service (PHS).[2] Within the PHS the National Institutes of Health (NIH) and the Alcohol, Drug Abuse, and Mental Health Administration (ADAMHA) allocate the largest percentage of federal funds for health-related research (Figure 2-4). Research funds in DHHS also are allocated to the Centers for Disease Control; the Health Care Financing

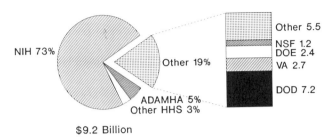

FIGURE 2-4 Source of federal support for health research and development for 1989. (Appendix Table A-1)

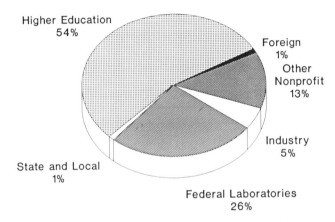

FIGURE 2-5 Distribution of federal health research funds for 1989.[2]

Administration; the Health Resources and Services Administration; the Food and Drug Administration; the Office of Health Research, Statistics, and Technology; and the Office of the Assistant Secretary for Health in the PHS. Other federal departments and agencies have budgets for health sciences research as well—most notably, the Departments of Defense, Energy, and Veterans Affairs, and the National Science Foundation (NSF) (Figure 2-4).

Unlike most other countries where government-sponsored research is conducted in government laboratories, two-thirds of federally sponsored health sciences research in the United States is conducted in institutions of higher education (colleges and universities), research organizations, and hospitals, and approximately one-quarter is performed in federal laboratories (Figure 2-5). Whereas the majority of industrial health sciences research is performed within corporate facilities, only a small fraction of federally sponsored research is performed in private industrial laboratories.[2]

The broad array of research sponsors and the decentralized nature of research efforts by thousands of individual health researchers are recognized widely as the key advantages to the U.S. approach to health research and as the means by which it has flourished over the past four decades. In this type of system the individual scientist is recognized as the most important element in determining scientific priorities. This has been accomplished primarily by scientists by serving on merit review panels and advisory groups. Currently, there are more than 2,000 nonfederal scientists serving on peer review study sections and advisory groups in the NIH alone.[6] Whereas the federal government along with other sponsors of research has been highly supportive of these peer review mechanisms and has provided financial resources for performing the research, many of the benefits of health research could not have been realized without a well-trained cadre of scientists.

Despite the success of the health research enterprise, the system has become stressed increasingly in recent years for many reasons. Most significant is the concern over growing federal debt and recent legislation attempting to reduce the huge annual federal budget outlays. Recent attempts to reduce federal deficits have increased the competition for scarce funds for all federally financed programs. Unfortunately, funds from states and private sector sources have been unable to compensate for the slower growth of available federal funds, especially support for fundamental health sciences research. The increasing competition among worthy projects has required making difficult choices, often resulting in concessions to short-term needs rather than longer-term investments.

This study committee was created out of a concern that these short-term choices have helped create an imbalance in the support of research projects, personnel, and the facilities and equipment needed for research. The committee examined the allocation policies of the primary sponsors of health research and the contributions to the scientific decision-making process by all concerned parties. This chapter overviews the funding of health research by the various sponsors and reviews policies affecting the allocation of these resources. The subsequent chapters examine more closely the sources and uses of funds for talent development, research projects, facilities and equipment, and processes for matching scientific priorities with political and fiscal realities.

FEDERAL SUPPORT FOR HEALTH SCIENCES R&D

NIH and ADAMHA

Before World War II nearly all federally sponsored health research was conducted in the government's own laboratories. The precursor to NIH, the Laboratory of Hygiene (later renamed the Hygienic Laboratory), was established out of the Marine Hospital Service in 1887 and was designated the National Institute of Health in 1930. Its role was expanded over the following decade to include public health advisory functions. The National Cancer Act of 1937 empowered the Surgeon General to administer extramural grants-in-aid for cancer research and provide fellowships to train scientific personnel. The Public Health Service Act of 1944 made NIH a separate entity in the PHS and empowered NIH to support research on diseases other than cancer through extramural grant and fellowship programs. The NIH Research Grants Office, forerunner of the Division of Research Grants, was created in 1946 to administer a program of extramural awards.

In 1953 the PHS was reassigned to the newly created Department of Health, Education, and Welfare, and the scope of NIH's responsibilities began to change.[7] In 1956 the National Library of Medicine Act created the National Library of Medicine (NLM) out of the Armed Forces Medical Library, and the Health Research Facilities Act was passed the same year, authorizing a program of matching funds to be administered through NIH for constructing health sciences research facilities. Growing appropriations under this new NIH construction authority were responsible for the major research building projects that expanded the research infrastructure in the United States from the late 1950s to 1970.

In response to new scientific opportunities in the health sciences, Congress increased funding for scientific research dramatically between 1945 and 1970, when appropriations for NIH rose from $26 million to $4.8 billion in constant 1988 dollars* (Figure 2-6).[7] Congress also added numerous categorical institutes to NIH during that time, reflecting efforts of special interest groups to target research on specific organ groups and illnesses. However, the rate of growth in funding for health sciences research slowed after 1965 in the wake of increased expenditures for the domestic human service initiatives of the Johnson administration and the Vietnam War.[8]

Despite this declining rate of budgetary growth, NIH continued to expand its role in the health sciences and underwent various reorganizations during the 1960s and 1970s.[7] In 1967 the National Institute of Mental Health (NIMH) was removed from NIH and established as a separate bureau within the PHS. Following this, in 1973, the recently created National Institute of Alcohol Abuse and Alcoholism (NIAAA) and the National Institute of Drug Abuse (NIDA) were merged with NIMH to form the

---

*All constant dollar figures in this text use the biomedical R&D price index developed by the Commerce Department for NIH. Although there are minor differences between the deflators for the intramural and extramural indices, only the combined deflator is used for all calculations.

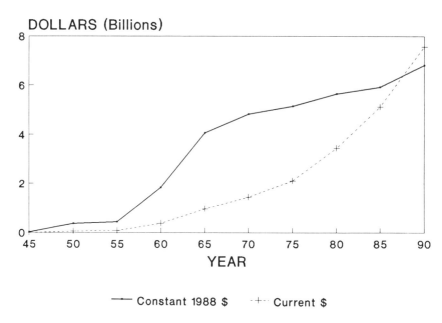

DOLLARS (Billions)

YEAR

⎯⎯ Constant 1988 $ ⁻⁺⁻ Current $

FIGURE 2-6   NIH appropriations from 1945 to 1990. Note: Constant dollars are calculated using the Biomedical Research and Development Price Index (BRDPI). (Appendix Table A-2)

ADAMHA. Also, during the 1970s, two institutes were elevated to bureau status within NIH, reflecting congressional emphasis on cancer and heart disease, and the National Institute of Aging was created because of an increasing desire to understand the aging process.

Inflationary pressures in the 1970s reduced the purchasing power of research funds, fostering the academic community's perception that the financial base of federal research support was eroding.[9] In response, the director of NIH advised Congress to stipulate the minimum number of new and competing research project grants that NIH would be required to support with its annual appropriations. This policy became known as "stabilization." Beginning in fiscal year 1981, NIH and ADAMHA were required to support 5,000 and 569 research project grants, respectively. Increasing target numbers were proposed for subsequent years but were negotiated between the administration and Congress during the annual federal budget process. Nonetheless, the appropriations for NIH grew steadily over the past decade (Figure 2-7). With the exception of 1982, NIH has realized a growth, after adjustments for inflation, of about 2 percent per year. Appropriations for ADAMHA, although they dropped in the early 1980s, had real growth in the research portion of the budget throughout the 1980s (Figure 2-8).[10] The research budgets for NIH and ADAMHA are covered in more detail in Chapter 4.

Over the past decade a variety of new laws and regulations have been enacted, affecting how federal research agencies carry out their missions and how they interact with industry, universities, and other extramural research institutions. For example, the Stevenson-Wydler Act (P.L. 96-480), passed in 1980, mandated that all agencies with R&D budgets allocate 0.5 percent of their research funds to industry or universities for technology transfer. In 1980 the Small Business Patent and Procedure Act (P.L. 96-517) made it possible to transfer patent rights derived from federally supported research to small businesses, universities, and certain nonprofit organizations.

The Small Business Innovation Development Act of 1982 established a program to grant federal research funds to for-profit businesses by all federal agencies with more than $100 million budgets for R&D.[7] This legislation called for a phase-in of the program over 4 subsequent fiscal years—from 1983 to 1986. Currently, all federal agencies awarding extramural research funds must allocate 1.25 percent of their annual R&D appropriations through this program.

The Federal Technology Transfer Act (P.L. 99-502) of 1986 encouraged additional government-industry collaboration. This legislation promotes technology transfer by authorizing government laboratories to enter into

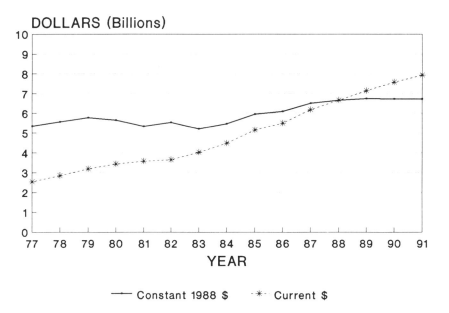

FIGURE 2-7 NIH appropriations from 1977 to 1991. Note: Figures for 1991 are derived from the President's proposed 1991 budget. (Appendix Table A-2)

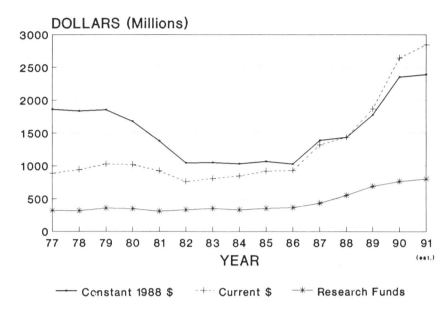

FIGURE 2-8   ADAMHA appropriations from 1977 to 1991. Note: Figures for 1991 are derived from the President's proposed 1991 budget. (Appendix Table A-2)

cooperative research and economic development agreements with other federal agencies, state and local governments, and for-profit and nonprofit organizations. Thus, companies now have unprecedented access to the research results from government laboratories upon which they can obtain exclusive licensing rights for development.[11]

Centers for Disease Control

The primary mission of the Centers of Disease Control (CDC) is to assist state and local health authorities and other health-related organizations in stemming the spread of communicable diseases, protecting the public from other diseases or conditions amenable to reductions, providing protection from certain environmental hazards, and improving occupational safety and health. Additionally, the CDC is responsible for licensing of clinical laboratories engaged in interstate commerce, for conducting foreign quarantine activities aimed at preventing the introduction of disease into the United States, and for developing scientific criteria for occupational health hazards. About nine-tenths of CDC's budget is allocated to the nonresearch portion of its mission, predominantly through block grants to states (Figure 2-9).

Of the $982 million appropriated to CDC in fiscal year 1989, only

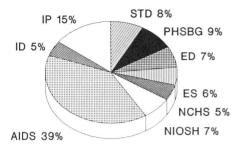

Percent of CDC Budget

FIGURE 2-9 Distribution of budget for the Centers for Disease Control for 1989.[14] (Key: IP = immunization program; STD = sexually transmitted diseases; PHSBG = preventive health services block grant; ED = environmental diseases; ES = epidemic services; NCHS = National Center for Health Statistics; NIOSH = National Institute for Occupational Safety and Health; AIDS = acquired immune deficiency syndrome; and ID = infectious diseases)

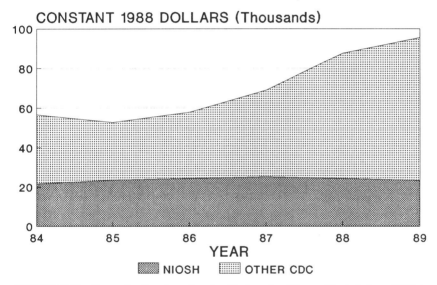

FIGURE 2-10 Research allocations for the Centers for Disease Control from 1984 to 1989. (Appendix Table A-3)

about 10 percent ($100.6 million) was obligated for health research. In constant 1988 dollars, research funds at CDC grew from $56.6 million to $95.5 million between 1984 and 1989 (Figure 2-10). Increases were greatest in fiscal years 1987 and 1988, when research funds grew by 18.8 and 26.8 percent, respectively, in constant dollars. These increases coincided directly with the increasing national emphasis on research into human immunodeficiency virus (HIV) infection.

The National Institute of Occupational Safety and Health (NIOSH) is the primary research arm of the CDC. NIOSH conducts research; develops criteria for occupational safety and health standards; and provides technical services to government, labor, and industry, including training in the recognition, avoidance, and prevention of unsafe or unhealthful working conditions and the proper use of adequate safety and health equipment. Through these various mechanisms, NIOSH tries to reduce the high economic and social costs associated with occupational illness and injury. Obligations for research funded by NIOSH grew only slightly between 1984 and 1987, and declined in the following 2 years (Figure 2-10). Of the $70.4 million appropriated to NIOSH for fiscal year 1989, $24.7 million was committed for research and about $10.1 million was obligated for training.*

The CDC has been a leader in the nation's efforts to prevent and control the spread of HIV infection, managing a comprehensive HIV prevention program that includes surveillance; epidemiologic and laboratory studies; and prevention through information, education, and risk reduction. Appropriations for AIDS activities for fiscal year 1989 were $382.3 million—39 percent of the CDC budget. The research portion of this allocation was $44.6 million for epidemiologic and laboratory studies to determine the natural history of the disease and to gain more knowledge about transmission of HIV. In fact, research funds allocated to other parts of CDC have grown much faster than those in NIOSH (Figure 2-10).

Another part of the CDC, the National Center for Health Statistics (NCHS), is responsible for collecting, maintaining, analyzing, and disseminating statistics on the health, illness, and disability of the U.S. population and on the impacts of these factors on the economy. Although this function is not classified under research, it is an ancillary service for epidemiological studies utilizing the data base. NCHS also is responsible for collecting nonhealth data on births, deaths, marriages, and divorces. For fiscal year 1989, $49 million dollars was appropriated to NCHS.

Office of the Assistant Secretary for Health

In the past, appropriations for the Office of Assistant Secretary for Health included funds for the National Center for Health Services Research and Health Care Technology Assessment (NCHSR). The center was the focal point within the federal government for research on the health care delivery system and examined problems in the organization, delivery, and financing of health care services. It was also within the center's purview to coordinate health services research in the PHS and to disseminate the

---

*There is a discrepancy between the NIOSH appropriations for research in the conference report from Congress ($60.5 million for fiscal year 1989) and the information received directly from CDC, which reported only $24.7 million.

findings of health services research to policy and decision makers in the public and private sectors.

The Reconciliation Act of 1986 established a program of medical care outcomes research to evaluate the appropriateness, necessity, and effectiveness of selected medical treatments and surgical procedures. Thus, Congress made available in the NCHSR's 1989 allocation $5.9 million from the Medicare trust funds, $3.9 million from the Federal Hospital Insurance Trust Fund, and $2.1 million from the Federal Supplementary Medical Insurance Trust Fund to fund outcomes research—funds that will support extramural research projects based on competitive peer review by NCHSR. These responsibilities have been transferred to the newly created Agency for Health Care Policy and Research (AHCPR).

Department of Veterans Affairs

Historically, the Department of Veterans Affairs (VA), previously known as the Veterans Administration, has provided health care to veterans through a network of 172 hospitals and centers nationwide. Approximately 130 of these units have medical trainees and about 100 have formal agreements with medical schools. The VA provides financial support for 8,350 residents and interns—nearly 13 percent of the trainees in the United States. Additionally, Congress appropriates R&D funds to the VA to conduct studies pertaining to veteran health or using veteran patient populations.

The VA R&D budget is a separate line item in the federal budget. In fiscal year 1989 the VA was appropriated $207.5 million for health sciences research; however, this does not reflect any increase over the last decade when measured in constant 1988 dollars (Figure 2-11). The VA research budget is divided into three major categories: (1) medical research, (2) rehabilitation research, and (3) health services R&D. The distribution among these categories for fiscal year 1988 was 85 percent, 11 percent, and 4 percent, respectively.

According to the VA, all R&D funds are peer reviewed, and 75 percent undergo a peer review process similar to investigator-initiated research project grants (R01) in the PHS. In 1981 the VA awarded 100 percent of its approved grant applications. However, the number of awards fell from more than 700 in 1985 to 386 in 1988. For 1989 the VA was able to fund approximately 500 meritorious research projects—an award rate of about 41 percent (Richard J. Greene, personal communication).

Approximately 10 percent of the VA research budget is allocated for career development at all levels. This includes limited salary support for some levels of training for young physician investigators. Generally, salary support for established VA investigators is covered with nonresearch funds.

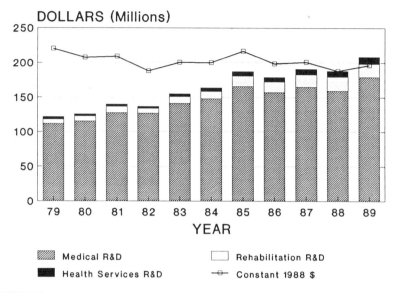

FIGURE 2-11   Research allocations for the Department of Veterans Affairs from 1979 to 1989. (Appendix Table A-4)

Eight percent of the research budget is directed toward VA Cooperative Studies (multihospital clinical trials).

The VA has several attributes that make it a good resource base for clinical research. First, patient recruitment for clinical investigations is easier for the VA than for NIH. Second, the costs for the standard medical care portion of clinical investigations are charged to health care delivery funds rather than research dollars; thus, only the marginal costs of the research consume research appropriations. The clinical trials conducted by the VA may have a far-reaching impact on research performed by other federal agencies. The VA also is exploring ways to enhance its position as a resource base for clinical investigations by more open cooperation with private industry.[12]

National Science Foundation

The NSF was founded as an independent government agency in 1950 to promote scientific progress through basic research in all fields of science and engineering. The NSF thus supports a broad spectrum of fields of science and has an equally broad portfolio of research support mechanisms. NSF awards comprise 28 percent of federal funding for basic research in academic institutions. Although its budget is only one-fourth that of NIH, the NSF plays an important role in setting science policy for the nation through the National Science Board.

As with NIH and ADAMHA, budget levels for NSF have risen steadily since its creation. However, in 1988 constant dollars NSF appropriations declined in the early 1980s and have returned to 1979 levels only recently (Figure 2-12).[13] The Reagan administration realized that basic research contributes significantly to U.S. competitiveness and therefore promised to commit the resources to NSF in order to double its budget in 5 years, but despite NSF budget requests of 19 percent increases for fiscal years 1988 and 1989, Congress increased appropriations by only 6 and 10 percent, respectively. NSF appropriations for fiscal year 1990 grew only modestly again to nearly $2.1 billion. Approximately $300 million, or 14 percent, of the 1989 appropriations were allocated to research and training related to the health sciences. Most of these funds are distributed through the Directorate of Biological, Behavioral, and Social Sciences (BBSS).

NSF's mission specifically excludes disease-related clinical research, which falls under the purview of NIH; therefore, NSF funds primarily are used for investigating basic biological processes that help shape the foundation for biomedical research. However, some funds are available for applied research, conferences and workshops, publication expenses, scientific equipment, libraries, and operation expenses of specialized research

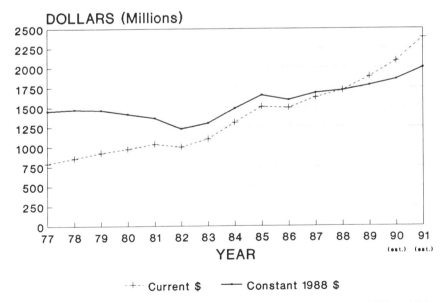

FIGURE 2-12 Appropriations for the National Science Foundation from 1977 to 1991. (Appendix Table A-5)

facilities. The current emphasis of NSF support is threefold: (1) continuing core support for basic research in all fields, (2) encouraging multidisciplinary projects, and (3) improving cooperation between academia and industry.

In 1988 the BBSS Directorate created the Division of Instrumentation and Resources to centralize its support for infrastructure and research resources. With regard to the health sciences, this division oversees the development of necessary biological software and data bases, genetic stock centers, and the acquisition of major specialized equipment for groups of investigators.

National Aeronautics and Space Administration

The National Aeronautics and Space Administration (NASA) has a small but highly specialized life sciences research program. The Office of Space Science and Applications at NASA spends approximately $75 million annually in its Life Sciences Division, of which about $37 million could be classified as health-related. This accounts for 0.4 percent of the total NASA budget, a level that has been maintained or lowered for the past decade.

The NASA biomedical research program is intended to support NASA's manned space programs. As the agency shifts from short-term space flights to more extended missions aboard the Space Station Freedom or to Mars, NASA will need to address specific questions relating to a microgravity environment, but because NASA has a very small life sciences budget, it must rely heavily on programs funded by other federal agencies.

Most of NASA's life science expenditures support intramural programs tailored to meet specific agency objectives. The agency does award small grants ($50 to $60 thousand) to investigators in the academic community. This, in effect, provides only partial support to extramural investigators but keeps an active community of scientists focusing on the problems associated with space travel.

Health Care Financing Administration

The primary mission of the Health Care Financing Administration (HCFA) is to manage the Medicare and Medicaid programs for health care payments, but the agency has a small research budget as well. Congress allocated $30 million to HCFA for research and demonstrations in fiscal year 1989.[14] These funds support a variety of studies on the Medicare and Medicaid populations and the health industry providing services to these populations. Issues that Congress wants HCFA to focus on include quality and access to health care; in-home and ambulatory care; special population needs, including those of minorities; and long-term care.

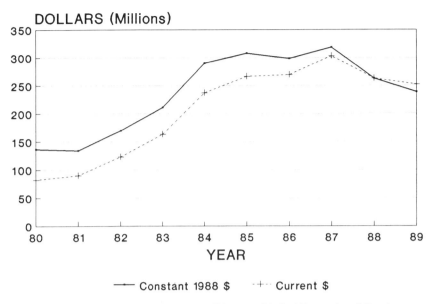

FIGURE 2-13 Research allocations for the U.S. Army Medical Research and Development Command from 1980 to 1989. (Appendix Table A-6)

Department of Defense

The Department of Defense (DOD) conducts health research vital to national security. Three branches conduct intramural and extramural health research: (1) the U.S. Army Medical Research and Development Command (USAMRDC), (2) the Directorate of Life Sciences in the Air Force Office of Scientific Research, and (3) the Life Sciences Programs Directorate of the Office of Naval Research.

Of the three branches, the USAMRDC receives the largest allocation of DOD funds for military health sciences research—about 80 percent of the total DOD health sciences research budget. In fiscal year 1989, $252 million was appropriated. When corrected to constant 1988 dollars, the USAMRDC budget grew from $136 million in 1980 to more than $318 million by 1987. However, this growth trend was reversed in 1988 and 1989, when the budget declined by 18 and 9 percent, respectively (Figure 2-13).

The USAMRDC conducts mission-oriented medical R&D designed to support the soldier in the field. More specifically, this program supports research on increasing manpower efficiency by improving instrumentation and new medical knowledge in the following areas: (1) military disease hazards, including infectious diseases, biological warfare defense, and AIDS;

(2) combat casualty care, including shock, wound healing, and craniofacial injuries; (3) medical chemical defense; and (4) army systems hazards. The Directorate of Life Sciences in the Air Force Office of Scientific Research has a much smaller health-related research budget than the US-AMRDC. In 1989, allocations for health research were only $17.1 million. These funds support research in several areas of neuroscience, experimental psychology, toxicology, visual and auditory psychophysics, radiation biology, and cardiovascular physiology.

The Office of Naval Research funds health research through the Life Sciences Programs Directorate. In fiscal year 1989 $24.4 million was allocated to biological and medical sciences and $11.5 million to cognitive and neural sciences. The 1990 budget request shows only slight growth for the biological and medical sciences—to $25.3 million—and $13.7 million for the cognitive and neural sciences.

Department of Energy

The Department of Energy (DOE) sponsors research related to the health effects of exposure to radiation and hazardous substances and has been a pioneer in the efforts to map the human genome. Most of the health research sponsored by DOE is conducted in the network of national laboratories under its direction. In 1989 and 1990, DOE allocated $218 million and $275 million to programs in biological and environmental research. However, its general life sciences program was allocated $45 million and $56 million for these past two years.

The largest portion of the life sciences program is mapping the human genome. Since both NIH and DOE have expertise in the necessary technology, a joint leadership plan is being implemented. DOE will develop the engineering technology and instrumentation crucial to the early stages of the project, and NIH will contribute through individual investigator work later. DOE allocations for this research endeavor have grown $18 million in 1989 to a proposed $46 million for fiscal year 1991. Both NIH and DOE have set up planning offices to coordinate the resources and efforts within the agencies. Additionally, the White House has created an interagency genome-coordination panel, under the authority of the White House Office of Science and Technology Policy, to work with NIH and DOE on project coordination. This precedent-setting interdepartmental effort will use the mechanisms outlined by the Federal Coordinating Council for Science, Engineering, and Technology (FCCSET).

INDUSTRY

Before World War II, industry funded more than half of all health sciences research in the United States.[3,4] After the war, industry's support, although still increasing, was outpaced by the investment of the federal government. Industry again is playing an increasingly important role in health sciences research, focusing primarily on product development. The types of industries engaged in health sciences R&D include biotechnology firms and manufacturers of pharmaceuticals, medical devices, and instrumentation. These industries tend to be much more research intensive than other U.S. corporations. Development and testing requirements for investigative new drugs or devices probably account for these larger R&D expenditures. Also, high levels of investment have been attributed in part to the commercial potential for genetically engineered products such as insulin.[15]

Individual corporations are reluctant to release proprietary data on their research programs. However, three aggregate measures of industrial investment related to biomedicine are available: (1) the NSF's Survey of Biotechnology Research and Development Activities in Industry, (2) the Annual Survey of the Pharmaceutical Manufacturers Association (PMA), and (3) a subset of companies included in *Business Week*'s "R&D Scoreboard." The criteria used to select companies for inclusion differ among surveys, and it is likely that some companies are included in more than one survey.

Although most corporate R&D is done "in house," industry relies heavily on university research programs for basic knowledge and scientific talent. However, pharmaceutical firms generally contract with clinicians in academic centers to test compounds in all phases of clinical trials. Corporate research focuses mainly on applied and developmental research rather than on disease-oriented research or fundamental basic biology. Shared interests in specific problems have helped create some industry-sponsored cooperative basic research programs located in universities.[16]

From the 1950s to the mid 1970s, industry focused its research programs on product development and relied largely on universities for basic research. By the 1970s policymakers and business people alike grew concerned that U.S. industry was losing its competitive edge in world markets, and this neglect of basic research was cited as a leading cause. Concern over foreign competition prompted U.S. industries to increase their investment in R&D markedly in the past decade. In 1977 industry spent approximately $20 billion on corporate R&D and somewhat over $100 million on research within universities. By 1986 their total R&D investment rose to nearly $60 billion internally and $600 million in university research.[14] In 1989 industry contributed about $9.3 billion to health sciences research, amounting to about 45 percent of the total national investment (Figure 2-2).[2]

Pharmaceutical Industry

The pharmaceutical industry increased expenditures for R&D by 16 percent in 1986 and 13 percent in 1987. Although the rate of increase slowed, it still exceeded the average industrial investment for R&D of 6 percent of gross income. Pharmaceutical firms also boast a high level of R&D expenditures in relation to sales, increasing from 11.6 percent in 1983 to 13.0 percent in 1987.

The distribution of R&D expenditures varies by company and type of research. The NSF reports that nearly 80 percent of industrial R&D is development, whereas basic research accounts for only 5 percent. The remaining 15 percent is categorized as applied research.[17] These estimates may not reflect R&D investment by the pharmaceutical industry correctly. However, according to one committee member, approximately one-third of a pharmaceutical firm's R&D investment is devoted to discovery and new product development, one-third is spent on existing product improvement and expansion of current business, and one-third is directed toward process improvement for defending current market shares of products. A large portion of pharmaceutical R&D is spent on clinical evaluation of drugs in phases I through IV (Table 2-1).

The pharmaceutical industry relies heavily on academia to provide new scientific talent. Scientific employment at U.S. pharmaceutical R&D facilities increased approximately 7 percent per year from 1983 to 1986. In 1986 the U.S. work force was 38,270 for PMA member firms, of which 24,500 were classified as scientific or professional.[18] While few companies provide training funds for predoctorates, several sponsor postdoctoral fellowships in their own research facilities. Also, the Pharmaceutical Manufacturers Association Foundation (PMAF), which is supported by dues from member firms, provides fellowships in pharmacology and related fields for postdoctoral trainees studying at academic institutions.

Biotechnology

Biotechnology is one subcategory of industrial biomedical R&D of particular importance to this committee. According to the Office of Technology Assessment (OTA), biotechnology is defined broadly as "any technique that uses living organisms (or parts of organisms) to make or modify products, to improve plants or animals, or to develop micro-organisms for specific uses."[19] However, traditional biotechnology, which has been employed throughout history for improving products, such as fermentation and animal husbandry, can be referred to as "old biotechnology." With the more

TABLE 2-1 Distribution of U.S. R&D Expenditures for Ethical Pharmaceuticals by Function, 1987 (dollars in millions)

Function	Amount	Percent
Clinical evaluation: phases I,II,III	$1,296.0	24.0
Biological screening and pharmacological testing	907.2	16.8
Synthesis and extraction	556.2	10.3
Pharmaceutical dosage formulation and stability testing	491.4	9.1
Toxicology and safety testing	448.2	8.3
Process development for manufacturing and quality control	507.6	9.4
Clinical evaluation: phase IV	237.6	4.4
Regulatory, IND and NDA preparation, submission and processing	194.4	3.6
Bioavailability studies	162.0	3.0
Other	599.4	11.1
TOTAL	5,400.0	100.0

Reprinted with permission. Pharmaceutical Manufacturers Association. 1989. Annual Survey Report of the U.S. Pharmaceutical Industry, 1987-1989. Washington, D.C.

recent understanding of genetics, recombinant DNA, cell fusion, and novel bioprocessing techniques have become known as "new biotechnology." Although the demarcation between old and new is somewhat cloudy, the committee focused only on the latter. (It also should be noted that not all biotechnology is in the realm of biomedical science.)

The federal government is the primary source of R&D funds for biotechnology; most funds come from NIH. NIH reported that nearly 22 percent or $1.02 billion of its 1988 R&D budget was allocated to research on developing biotechnology techniques or employing the technology. The size of the NIH investment in biotechnology reflects the importance of molecular genetics in biomedicine.

The OTA conducted two surveys of biotechnology firms in 1987. Of the 296 dedicated biotechnology firms contacted in the first survey, 63 (21 percent) were involved with human therapeutics and 52 (18 percent) were conducting R&D in diagnostics. In the second survey of 53 large, diversified companies investing in biotechnology, 20 were performing R&D in human therapeutics and diagnostics. Overall, OTA estimated that, as of

January 1988, 403 dedicated biotechnology firms and more than 70 major corporations were investing in biotechnology. OTA estimated further that the total investment by industry was between $1.5 and $2.0 billion per year.

The NSF surveyed corporations engaged in biotechnology research as a pilot study for future investigation of industrial R&D in emerging technologies.[20] In 1986 and 1987 the NSF sent questionnaires to firms expected to spend at least $1 million annually on biotechnology R&D. A total of 54 firms responded to both surveys—a total estimated to account for half of all industrial investment in biotechnology R&D.[21] These 54 companies increased their R&D investments by 20 percent in 1985 but by only 16 and 12 percent, respectively, in 1986 and 1987. Although these firms showed a slowing rate of growth for R&D investment, their expenditures as a percent of sales continued to surpass those of industry overall. The NSF estimated that industry invested $1.4 billion in biotechnology R&D in 1987.

General Trends

From 1985 through 1987, *Business Week* reported both sales and R&D expenditures for 38 health care companies in its R&D scoreboard. These firms have continued to increase their rate of investment in R&D—from 12 percent in 1986 to 16 percent in 1987. These rates exceeded industrial averages by 2 percent in 1986 and 9 percent in 1987. In addition, the health care firms' ratio of R&D investment to sales surpassed the average industrial ratio by more than 4 percent.

The NSF survey estimated that the biotechnology industry spent $1.4 billion on R&D in 1987 and that pharmaceutical manufacturers invested nearly $5.4 billion in the same year.[11] This suggests that industry's contribution to biomedical R&D is comparable to the total NIH budget. NIH staff members have estimated that industry is the most rapidly growing sector of health R&D and that the aggregate industrial investment in biomedical R&D has exceeded the NIH budget since 1982. In fact, the PMA has reported that the combined total R&D expenditures of its member firms exceeded the NIH budget in 1989.[18]

Recently, it appears that the growth of industrial investment in R&D has begun to level off. This slower growth has been attributed to mergers that force corporations to cut costs, to economic troubles in some industries, and to other pressures to show short-term profits.[14] Additionally, a reduction in tax credits for incremental increases in R&D investment may have caused some firms to trim their R&D expenditures. The NSF and PMA surveys suggest that growth of industrial investment in biomedical R&D has plateaued. This could indicate that the field of biotechnology has begun to mature or that firms engaged in biomedical R&D are not immune to the economic pressures facing all U.S. corporations.

Legislation Affecting Corporate R&D

In the past decade the federal government helped industry strengthen its associations with universities. For example, the NSF developed special research centers to foster collaboration between universities and corporations.[11] In addition, the antitrust law was relaxed so as to permit companies within the same industry to form nonprofit research consortia, such as Sematech.

The 1981 Economic Recovery Tax Act provided a tax credit for incremental increases in R&D spending to foster additional investment and stimulate technology transfer. In a recent report, the General Accounting Office estimates that the tax credit stimulated between $1 billion and $2.5 billion of additional R&D between 1981 and 1985. However, the cost was estimated to be $7 billion in foregone tax revenues.[22] While these costs seem high, the societal benefits derived from the research may be much higher.

The law expired in 1985 but was renewed in 1986. However, the renewal trimmed the tax credit from 25 to 20 percent of investment and added restrictions to the types of research that qualified for the credit. Also, the 1986 renewal included a 20 percent credit for industry-supported research conducted at universities and other academic institutions.

The credits, set to expire in 1988, again were extended through 1989 and although companies still could receive a 20 percent tax credit, they had to reduce the R&D expenses they deducted on their tax returns by an amount equal to half of the earned credit.[23] New bills introduced into the House and Senate continue this provision. President Bush, who favors making the tax credit permanent, is supporting a provision for companies to subtract 100 percent of the tax credit value from their declared R&D expenses. The administration also would like to allow start-up companies to carry earned credits forward 15 years, for these companies generally do not earn taxable profits in their early years and therefore cannot benefit from the present law.

The Technology Transfer Act of 1986 was intended to facilitate more active collaboration between industry and federal agencies involved in R&D. Although this legislation was intended in part to respond to the steadily rising costs of health care, the legislation actually dampened enthusiasm for these collaborations between some corporations and NIH. Pharmaceutical firms are displeased particularly because of the government's insistence on imposing price controls for 10 years after development on new drugs developed cooperatively.

University-Industry Cooperation

In 1986 industry contributed approximately 5 percent to overall support for academic research. Despite increasing academic research funding from industry since then, industry investment is not expected to exceed 7 to 8 percent of university research budgets. The mechanisms of this industrial support for academic research span the spectrum, from small, unrestricted gifts and contract research to highly organized cooperative ventures.

Many issues are involved when cooperative ventures between universities (or government) and industry are established. Differences exist between the cultures of corporations and universities, the most notable being freedom of information. For instance, in-house corporate research is proprietary information, but similar secrecy and publication constraints in a university setting can threaten the very essence of university freedom. Despite these differences, however, a number of cooperative ventures have succeeded in the past decade. Reconciliation between the goals and expectations of industry and academe has been and remains crucial to their success. When successful, these cooperatives provide a unique technology transfer mechanism, one of the federal government's key policies for increasing U.S. economic competitiveness.

An example of successful industrial support of university research is the Monsanto Corporation's collaborative research effort with Washington University on the peptides and proteins that regulate cellular function and communication. Monsanto initiated the arrangement in 1982 to support research in an area in which it did not have in-house expertise. The firm provides a pool of funds for grants to Washington University faculty, with 30 percent allocated to basic research and 70 percent to projects that may result eventually in the development of commercial products. Research results are made public, and Washington University holds patents on products created by the research. Monsanto reserves both the right to view results for 30 days before submission for publication and the right of first refusal for exclusive licensing to develop products. Under this arrangement, Monsanto is expected to have provided the university with $62 million for research by 1990.[16]

NONPROFIT ORGANIZATIONS

During the nineteenth and the first half of the twentieth centuries, private nonprofit foundations constituted a primary source of funds for health sciences research. Many early foundations were established to benefit particular institutions or to address specific social or health problems. These foundations' assets were derived generally from an individual's or family's gifts. During the twentieth century, voluntary health agencies, which are referred to also as operating foundations, have proliferated. Additionally, a special type of nonprofit organization—the medical research organization—has developed, such as the Howard Hughes Medical Institute.

Each of these types of organizations differs in its mission, governance, and mechanisms of support. Although these organizations comprise a limited portion of health sciences research support, they are vital to the nation's research enterprise because of their flexibility and their dedication to curing human disease and suffering. The NIH estimated that private nonprofit organizations contributed about $700 million (or about 4.3 percent of the total), to health R&D in 1988.[2] However, this figure probably underestimates the role of philanthropy in health sciences research by excluding endowed professorships and donations for facilities and equipment. Another estimate has placed philanthropy at nearly one-quarter of a typical institution's budget for biomedical R&D.[4]

Foundations

In the early 1900s the philosophy of foundation philanthropy began to change, becoming less restrictive as broad charters were given to the boards of directors of such newly formed foundations as the Rockefeller and Russell Sage Foundations and the Carnegie Corporation of New York.[4] These charters allowed the directors to focus their foundation's philanthropy in ways they believed would provide the greatest social benefit rather than at specific problems. At the same time, community foundations were beginning to form in cities around the United States. Unlike independent foundations, these community foundations relied (and continue to rely) on charitable contributions.

Tax law changes in the mid 1930s allowed corporations to deduct charitable contributions and fostered the formation of corporate foundations to serve as the primary philanthropic arm of companies. Presently, there are more than 400 company-sponsored foundations actively involved in grant support, and they provide more than $2 billion per year to all scientific areas, including the health sciences.

Since World War II, federal investment in health sciences research has eclipsed that of foundations, but foundations still play a vital role in the research enterprise, augmenting federal funding for health sciences research. However, some foundations that support health-related activities may not support research directly; rather, they support talent development or facilities. Also, some foundations that previously supported research no longer do so. Nonetheless, foundations, in general, have provided crucial support in filling gaps in the research agenda that have not been addressed appropriately or profitably by government or industry.

Currently, private foundations provide a great variety of support mechanisms for health sciences research. Few of these foundations conduct in-house research, most believing that extramural research provides the most efficient use of funds. Common types of foundation support include individual research project grants, predoctoral and postdoctoral fellowships, equipment grants, publication expenses, special library collections grants, and sponsorship of conferences or workshops. Large, independent foundations contributing to health sciences research include but are not limited to the following: the Lucille P. Markey Trust, the Pew Charitable Trusts, the Duke Endowment, the Commonwealth Fund, the Alfred P. Sloan Foundation, the John A. Hartford Foundation, the Henry J. Kaiser Family Foundation, the Robert Wood Johnson Foundation, the John D. and Catherine T. MacArthur Foundation, and the Andrew W. Mellon Foundation.[4]

The mechanisms for priority setting vary among foundations—company sponsored as well as independent. In some instances, funding decisions are made through personal contacts or because of interest in a specific disorder. Large, independent foundations may form advisory committees to determine areas of emphasis; proposals also may be subjected to a peer review process similar to that used by NIH. Smaller foundations may not plan program initiatives but rather may fund the best unsolicited proposals received in a given time period. The extent of foundation support for health sciences research varies from year to year, depending on the relative timing of costly initiatives. Also, company-sponsored foundations frequently restrict support in communities in which the company has operations and in programs that may affect its employees directly. Several committee members believe that corporate charity is becoming more closely tied to individual employee charitable giving, with corporate donations often matching the employee's contributions. This diminishes the size of corporate gifts to academic institutions for research purposes.

Tax laws and the economic environment affect foundation contributions to all areas, including the health sciences. Until 1969 there were few specific federal regulations pertaining to foundations. Modifications to the Internal Revenue Code in that year, however, changed the rules regarding organizations classified as private foundations by federal tax law. Included in the changes were restrictions on self-dealing and limitations on business ownership. Now, all foundations with assets exceeding $5,000 must file an annual report with the IRS, listing all of the principal officers of the foundation, its total assets and investments, and every grant made in that year.

Prior to the Tax Reform Act of 1976, a foundation's annual giving requirements were based on whichever was greater: adjusted net income or a variable percentage of the market value of investment assets. The 1976 act fixed the giving requirements at 5 percent of market value assets or net income, and it eliminated the variable percentage method. Private foundations were being charged a 4 percent excise tax on their net investment until 1978, when the law reduced the tax rate to 2 percent. The Economic Recovery Tax Act of 1981 changed the giving requirements again to equal a flat 5 percent of market value of assets per year. These tax law changes have contributed to the growth of foundation giving in recent years.

Since giving requirements are tied directly to the market value of foundation assets, the economy has a significant effect on total giving. In periods of high inflation, such as that experienced in the late 1970s, foundations actually lost assets when measured in constant dollars. However, the bull markets and low inflation rates of the 1980s helped increase the value of foundation assets and subsequently increased contributions to health research.

Voluntary Health Agencies

Voluntary health agencies (often referred to as operating foundations) are private charities supported primarily by public donations. There are now perhaps as many as 200 national and regional organizations actively supporting health research. Many of these organizations were founded by the families and friends of individuals suffering from a particular disease.

These voluntary health agencies, such as the American Cancer Society and the American Heart Association, play critically important roles in advancing their areas of interest. With activities that include public awareness and education, patient referrals, continuing education for health professionals, grants for research and training, and lobbying to increase federal funding for disease-specific research. However, it should be noted that not all disease-specific organizations support research, and of those that do, most do not conduct in-house research.

The six largest voluntary health agencies (in terms of revenues) are, in descending order, the American Cancer Society, the American Heart Association, the March of Dimes-Birth Defects Foundation, the Muscular Dystrophy Association, the National Easter Seal Society, and the American Lung Association. These six organizations reported combined expenditures for disease-related research of more than $250 million in 1988.* Since these organizations rely on voluntary contributions, they are not able to make long-term commitments to research efforts. However, they are effective in responding rapidly to new research initiatives and in providing resources to scientists to develop new lines of investigation.

The voluntary health agencies also can play a very critical role in the

---

*Figures were obtained from 1988 annual reports.

early stages of many individuals' scientific career development. Through funding mechanisms such as fellowships and career development awards, these organizations attract young researchers to a specific field and provide them with research funding before they are able to compete successfully for federal support. Grant awards from these organizations commonly range between $20,000 and $50,000.

Voluntary health agencies also act as lobbyists for increases in disease-specific funds for NIH. These organizations increase public awareness of the need to fight particular diseases and solicit grass-roots support for more federal research funds, and they also have been very influential in establishing new institutes at NIH.

Medical Research Organizations

Medical research organizations (MRO), such as the Howard Hughes Medical Institute (HHMI) and the J. David Gladstone Foundation Laboratories for Cardiovascular Disease, conduct medical research in conjunction with hospitals. By law, these types of organizations must spend 3.5 percent of their endowments on medical research annually. The Gladstone Foundation is a relatively small medical research organization with assets estimated at $118 million and is affiliated with the University of California at San Francisco.

On the other extreme, the largest MRO is HHMI with assets in excess of $6 billion. In recent years HHMI has become the largest single private nonprofit contributor to biomedical research. Currently, HHMI's total investment in biomedical research is comparable to the budget of a small institute within NIH, with expenditures totaling $238.4 million in 1989. The trustees have designed the institute's program to complement NIH activities within a few selected areas of research: cell biology and regulation, genetics, immunology, neuroscience, and structural biology. A 10 member medical advisory board has ultimate responsibility for the quality of the research program, whereas scientific review boards composed of scientists in each of the five areas oversee work in their respective fields. Although the institute is sufficiently large to make a major contribution, it does not seek to replace the central role of NIH in any field.

HHMI traditionally has established large laboratories with a core group of investigators in universities and hospitals around the United States to facilitate interaction with the larger research community. Investigators are appointed for fixed terms of 3 to 7 years, with full funding provided for faculty and technician salaries as well as research expenses. Investigator productivity is evaluated through research conferences, annual progress reports, and site visits.

By mid 1988 HHMI employed approximately 180 investigators and a

1,350-member support staff in 30 sites. In order to expand the number of host institutions, HHMI recently began to support individual investigators rather than multi-investigator laboratories. The institute plans to support approximately 250 investigators and 2,000 support staff in at least 40 sites within a few years.

HHMI has undertaken a broad program to strengthen science education from the precollege to the postdoctoral stages. The Institute is funding a study by the Commission of Life Sciences of the National Academy of Sciences that is examining the curricula and teaching of high school biology. The new HHMI Undergraduate Science Education Program awards grants to strengthen science education and research in private undergraduate colleges. Begun in 1988, the program is intended to increase the number of students, especially minorities and women, pursuing careers in the biomedical sciences. In 1988 HHMI awarded $30.4 million to 44 colleges, including 10 historically black colleges. Expansion of this program in 1989 granted $61 million to 51 undergraduate colleges affiliated with research universities and other doctorate-granting institutions.

The graduate science education program funds several levels of graduate training. For instance, doctoral fellowships in the biological sciences (60 per year) provide predoctoral students with a stipend and cost-of-education allowance for 3 to 5 years; medical Student Research Training Fellowships (up to 60 per year) are modeled after HHMI's Research Scholars Program, supporting students for a year of research training at any U.S. academic or research institution. The Research Resources Program funds development of institutional infrastructures related to graduate research and education. The resources program may provide support in the following areas: courses and symposia concerned directly with HHMI areas of interest, replenishment of biological stocks and materials, and genetic analysis projects that complement the HHMI human genome data base.

SUMMARY AND CONCLUSIONS

The committee concluded that health research is supported by a diverse, yet interlocking network of federal agencies, industry, and private nonprofit organizations. Of these, the federal government is the single largest sponsor of health research in the U.S. Of the $71 billion the federal government will invest in R&D during fiscal year 1991, nearly $10 billion will be health related. Contributions by health-oriented corporations are roughly equal in magnitude, but devoted largely to product application developments rather than fundamental discovery research. Contributions by private nonprofit sponsors favor fundamental discovery research, generally in somewhat restricted fields of interest, but represent only about 4 to 5 percent of the total U.S. investment in health research.

In light of this investment and the continuing budget limitations, the scientific community must reexamine its resource base to improve its effectiveness and efficiency. Federally sponsored health research by the various agencies is generally mission oriented. NIH and ADAMHA are the primary agencies that disburse federal health research funds for investigation into fundamental biological discovery, but the committee emphasizes that all health research expands the boundaries of knowledge.

Although industry has been playing an increasingly important role in health research, focusing primarily on product development, it relies heavily on university research programs for basic scientific knowledge and talent. Cooperative ventures between universities (or government) and industry provide a unique mechanism for sharing knowledge and technology transfer, a central policy of the federal government for increasing U.S. economic competitiveness.

Foundations, voluntary health agencies, and other nonprofit organizations have played a very important role in sponsoring health research. The committee believes that these organizations have been particularly helpful in providing crucial support in filling gaps in the nation's research agenda and sponsoring new initiatives. Although the federal government rapidly eclipsed the investment by these organizations following World War II, they have continued to supply a steady stream of research dollars. These funds are used for individual research projects, supporting career development awards in specific research fields, equipment, facilities, and various programs of knowledge dissemination. The committee anticipates that these organizations will continue to provide support for the health sciences.

REFERENCES

1. National Science Foundation. 1989. Science and Technology Resources: Funding and Personnel. Publication No. 89-300. Washington, D.C.
2. U.S. Department of Health and Human Services; Public Health Service. 1989. NIH Data Book 1989. Publication No. 89-1261. Bethesda, Md.: National Institutes of Health.
3. Ginzberg, E. and A.B. Dutka. 1989. The Financing of Biomedical Research. Baltimore: The Johns Hopkins University Press.
4. Boniface, Z.E. and R.W. Rimel. 1987. U.S. Funding of Biomedical Research. Philadelphia: The Pew Charitable Trusts.
5. Bush, V. 1945. Science–The Endless Frontier, A Report to the President on a Program for Postwar Scientific Research. Washington, D.C.: Office of Scientific Research and Development. (Reprinted by the National Science Foundation, May 1980.)
6. U.S. Department of Health and Human Services; Public Health Service. 1986. DRG Peer Review Trends; Member Characteristics: DGR Study Sections, Institute Review Groups, Advisory Councils and Boards, 1976-1986. Bethesda, Md.: National Institutes of Health.
7. U.S. Department of Health and Human Services; Public Health Service. 1989 NIH Almanac. Publication No. 89-5. Bethesda, Md.: National Institutes of Health.

8.   Strickland, S.P. 1972. Politics, Science, and Dread Disease: A Short History of United States Medical Research Policy. Cambridge, Mass.: Harvard University Press.

9.   Seggel, R. L. 1985. Stabilizing the Funding of NIH and ADAMHA Research Project Grants. Washington, D.C.: National Academy Press.

10. U.S. Department of Health and Human Services; Public Health Service. 1989. ADAMHA Data Source Book 1988. Rockville, Md.: Alcohol, Drug Abuse, and Mental Health Administration.

11. U.S. Congress; Office of Technology Assessment. 1988. New Developments in Biotechnology: U.S. Investment in Biotechnology–Special Report. OTA-BA-360. Washington, D.C.: U.S. Government Printing Office.

12. Institute of Medicine. 1989. Government and Industry Collaboration in Biomedical Research and Education. Washington, D.C.: National Academy Press.

13. National Science Foundation. 1987. Report on Funding Trends and Balance of Activities: National Science Foundation 1951-1988. NSF 88-3. Washington, D.C.

14. U.S. House of Representatives. 1989. Report of the House of Representatives Appropriations Subcommittee for the Departments of Labor, Health and Human Services, and Education, and Related Agencies Appropriations Bill, 1989, Report No. 100-689. Washington, D.C.

15. Boniface, Z.E. U.S. Funding for Biomedical Research: An Update. Background paper prepared for this study committee.

16. National Academy of Sciences; Government-University-Industry Research Roundtable. 1986. New Alliances and Partnerships in American Science and Engineering. Washington, D.C.: National Academy Press.

17. National Science Foundation. 1988. The Science and Technology Resources of Japan: A Comparison with the United States. NSF 88-318. Washington, D.C.

18. Pharmaceutical Manufacturers Association. 1989. Annual Survey Report of the U.S. Pharmaceutical Industry, 1987-89. Washington, D.C.

19. U.S. Congress; Office of Technology Assessment. 1984. Commercial Biotechnology: An International Analysis. OTA-BA-218. Washington, D.C.

20. National Science Foundation. 1987. Biotechnology Research and Development Activities in Industry: 1984 and 1985. NSF 87-311. Washington, D.C.

21. National Science Foundation. 1988. Science Resource Highlights: Industrial Biotechnology R&D Increased an Estimated 12 Percent in 1987 to $1.4 Billion. NSF 88-306. Washington, D.C.

22. U.S. General Accounting Office. 1989. The Research Tax Credit Has Stimulated Some Additional Research Spending. Report number GAO/GGD-89-114. Washington, D.C.

23. Science. 1989. Fate of R&D tax credit uncertain. Vol. 243, March 31, P. 1659.

3
Setting Federal Science and Technology Priorities

Defense, health, foreign affairs, space, commerce, and transportation all contain elements of science and technology. The science and technology issues in these various sectors are affected increasingly by governmental processes in the administration and Congress and are evaluated and judged on their importance to the larger governmental mission.[1] Federal science and technology priority setting is a complex procedure involving the President, Congress, the scientific community, the public, and their many special interest groups (Figure 3-1).

Federal priorities are often reflected in the amount of funds allocated to each portion of the budget. In recent years there have been enormous fiscal pressures on all federally financed programs because of growing federal debt. These budget constraints have become particularly acute since the enactment of the Balanced Budget and Emergency Deficit Control Act of 1985, also known as the Gramm-Rudman-Hollings Act (GRH), which has sought to reconcile annual federal revenues and outlays in a concerted effort to balance the federal budget by 1992. Thus, the committee feels that it is important to be fully aware of the organizational structure and processes of the federal health sciences establishment as well as the external forces that are shaping the federal budget.

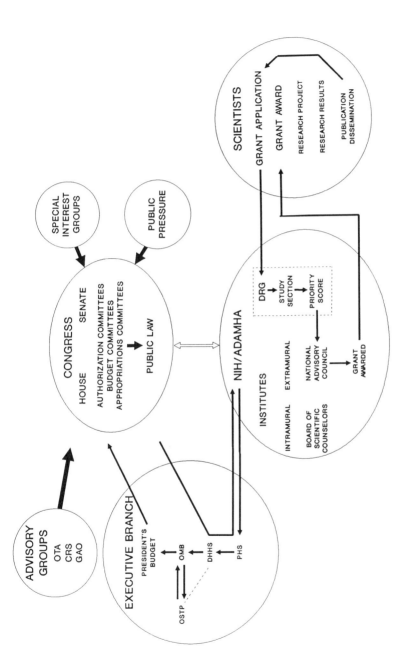

FIGURE 3-1 Schematic diagram of federal budgeting, priority setting, and granting of research funds.

SCIENCE AND TECHNOLOGY ADVICE TO GOVERNMENT

Presidential Science and Technology Advice

A formalized system for science advice to the President dates back to the 1940s—to President Roosevelt's administration during World War II. After the war President Truman, with strong encouragement from congressional leaders, sought advice in organizing a body to provide scientific advice to the executive office. Beginning in 1951, the Science Advisory Committee to the President was located in the Office of Defense Mobilization. The launching of Sputnik focused public attention on the American scientific establishment, and in 1957 President Eisenhower created the President's Science Advisory Committee (PSAC) and designated its chairman as his special assistant for science and technology.[2] Although PSAC was concerned primarily with the military aspects of scientific research, it laid the groundwork for scientific advisors for later administrations. PSAC was sanctioned officially by executive order in the Kennedy, Johnson, and Nixon administrations. During these administrations, PSAC's role was defined by the incumbent President and generally emphasized military weapons evaluation, although in the 1960s PSAC's scope expanded to include civilian scientific endeavors as well.

During the Nixon administration, PSAC was regarded highly by the scientific/technical community; however, the internal working structure of the Nixon White House and the various departments and agencies did not share this view.[3] Much of the work by the Nixon PSAC was self-initiated, and PSAC thus was criticized for meddling in the internal affairs of government departments. PSAC was abolished by President Nixon in 1973, apparently because of growing divergences between PSAC and presidential-level viewpoints.[4]

Congress sought to eliminate the problems experienced with PSAC in providing scientific advice to the President by passing the Science Advisory Act of 1976 (P.L. 94-282). This legislation made the head of the Office of Science and Technology Policy (OSTP) equivalent to the heads of other executive offices, such as the director of the Office of Management and Budget (OMB) or the Chairman of the Council of Economic Advisors. With this act Congress attempted to improve the science advisor's access to the President and avoid the political pitfalls experienced by PSAC by mandating specific functions for OSTP that would be subject to congressional oversight.[5] Congress also attempted to provide OSTP with sufficient staff to deal with a broad spectrum of issues, without diluting its effectiveness. Lastly, Congress sketched out in the act the elements of a national science and technology policy, identifying 10 areas of national importance that defined the charge to the science advisor. The law broadly states the charge to the science advisor: "The primary function of the Director of OSTP is to provide, within the Executive Office of the President, advice on the scientific, engineering, and technological aspects of issues that require attention at the highest levels of government."

The Science Advisory Act included provisions for an Office of Science and Technology Policy, with a director and as many as four associate directors appointed with the advice and consent of the Senate. Although Congress authorized four associate directors, no more than two of these positions were ever filled at any one time until this year. Also, an adequate staff is necessary to address the broad scope of responsibilities assigned to the science and technology advisor and the associate directors of OSTP. The number of full-time permanent staff in OSTP has declined from 23 in the late 1970s to 11 in early 1989. Moreover, Congress has severely limited the use of "detailees" or borrowed staff from executive agencies and governmental laboratories, who in the past have provided necessary staffing and expertise that is not covered adequately by the budget.

Congress expected OSTP to become a major policy arm of government. Despite Congress's good intentions, it has been unable to guarantee that the President or his close advisors will receive information on or give attention to the scientific implications of national policy issues. In the years since the Science Advisory Act was passed, science advice to the President by the director of OSTP has been dealt with in varying ways by the Ford, Carter, and Reagan administrations. The President's science advisor has a dual role as an individual member of the White House staff (often designated Assistant to the President) and the head of a policy office in the Executive Office of the President. However, the relationship between the science advisor and the President depends largely upon the advisory structure and management style within the White House. Some presidents rely on cabinet members as their policy advisors, whereas others use White House advisors to guide their administration. Also, the science advisor's effectiveness is judged by the importance of the scientific issues dealt with by the President as well as the relatedness of science policies to the national agenda. However, a poor relationship with the President may weaken the science and technology advisory capabilities of OSTP.

A 1988 report by the National Academy of Sciences entitled *Science and Technology Advice in the White House* suggested the optimal functions and qualifications of a science and technology advisor and suggested changes in the organization of OSTP.[6] The science and technology advisor to the President can fulfill this vital role through activities that shape federal science policy: (1) formulating policy pertaining to the nation's R&D efforts, (2) recruiting senior-level personnel to executive positions in agencies with science and technology functions, (3) evaluating R&D budgets, in cooperation with the OMB, (4) coordinating R&D management among the various departments and agencies, and (5) advising the President on the implications of international negotiations involving science and technology. In order to provide independent and objective counsel, the Academy report indicated that the science and technology advisor must have certain attributes. These include developing a relationship of trust, mutual respect, and open communication with the President; forming a wide-ranging set of high-quality study groups to focus on important questions; tapping into the scientific community and its institutions in an ongoing, broad-based way, both in government and outside of it; and earning a reputation for integrity without having preconceived answers to technical or policy questions.

Ad hoc committees and advisory consultants can play an important role in providing advice to the administration as well. The director of OSTP can readily call upon distinguished members of the scientific and lay community to serve in a short-term advisory capacity by authority of the Intergovernmental Personnel Act. This allows the administration to receive timely information on science and technology issues vital to national interests. Likewise, ad hoc or standing committees can be established to confront those issues needing urgent attention.

In the Reagan Administration the White House Science Council (WHSC) was established by George Keyworth under the authority of the Federal Advisory Committees Act in 1981. The WHSC was a bipartisan group of nongovernmental scientists and engineers from academia and industry that reported to the director of OSTP. The WHSC met with the President and other senior members of the Administration to review issues identified by the council or the director of OSTP. After an 8-year hiatus, the committee advisory function previously performed by PSAC was performed by the WHSC in the Reagan White House, the primary difference being that the chairman of the Council was not the science advisor to the President. Insofar as neither PSAC or the WHSC are established by statute, each President and/or his science advisor has the authority to establish an outside advisory mechanism that best suits the administration.

In the present administration the director of OSTP, D. Allan Bromley, has created a President's Council of Advisors on Science and Technology (PCAST) that will replace the WHSC from the previous administration.* In much the same fashion as the original PSAC, the director of OSTP will be the chairman of PCAST, and the members will be nongovernmental presidential appointees from a broad spectrum of science and engineering

---

*PCAST members are Norman E. Borlaug, Solomon J. Buchsbaum, Charles L. Drake, Ralph E. Gomery, Bernadine Healy, Peter W. Likins, Thomas E. Lovejoy, Walter E. Massey, John P. McTague, Daniel Nathans, David Packard, and Harold T. Shapiro.

fields. In effect, PCAST will provide vital science and engineering advice to the President through OSTP.

The Federal Coordinating Council on Science, Engineering, and Technology (FCCSET) was authorized by the National Science and Technology Policy, Organizations, and Priorities Act of 1986 to evaluate interagency research efforts. FCCSET is composed of the director of OSTP and one representative of each of the following 13 federal agencies: the Departments of Agriculture, Commerce, Defense, Health and Human Services, Housing and Urban Development, Interior, State, Energy, Veterans Affairs, and Transportation, the National Science Foundation (NSF), Environmental Protection Agency, and the National Aeronautics and Space Administration. Under FCCSET various committees composed of appropriate high-level federal agency representatives can be established to provide a direct link among governmental agencies and can serve as a coordinating mechanism. Under the chairmanship of the science and technology advisor, FCCSET can bring together cabinet officials and agency directors to address regulatory, administrative, or budgetary issues of mutual interest. Examples of such efforts include the biotechnology writing group, which answered directly to the White House Economic Policy Council via the science advisor and, more recently, the interagency genome-coordinating council.[7]

The effectiveness of future science and technology advisors to the President will depend largely on the issues that will be confronted, scientific interest and priorities of the President and his staff, the professional relationships in the Executive Office of the President, and the expertise and breadth of knowledge of the advisor and his staff. Thus, the committee concluded that appropriate mechanisms are in place for providing effective science advice to the President.

Congressional Science and Technology Advice

Since the agenda for science and technology ultimately is set by Congress through its authorizing, budgeting, and appropriating activities, advice to Congress and its key science committees is equally important. There are many advisory bodies that provide science and technology advice to Congress. The most public method is by congressional hearing. Experts from universities, industry, and governmental agencies frequently are called upon to testify before congressional committees on issues relating to science and technology policies.

Congressional aides also are an important resource for science and technology information. With staff terms lasting longer than many member terms and with a high ratio of advanced degrees among staff members, there is a cadre of scientific support personnel within Congress. Aides assist members in developing information germane to potential legislation, either by researching issues themselves or identifying speakers for hearings. These aides also are helpful in drafting legislation and preparing member presentations on issues relating to pending legislation. Finally, staff as well often gather information from other congressional staff or help the member garner support for legislation.

Major research support systems also assist Congress in developing science policy. The Library of Congress maintains a staff in the Science Policy Research Division of the Congressional Research Service (CRS). This group may be called upon to provide information or conduct detailed studies on issues affecting science and technology policy. The CRS maintains a professional staff of 35 to 40 individuals to provide objective nonpartisan reports at the request of congressional members. Experts also are contacted by phone and review report drafts.

Another major science policy support resource is the Office of Technology Assessment (OTA). This office was established by Congress in 1972 to conduct in-depth analyses and formulate recommendations for potential legislation, and it frequently tackles major science policy issues. OTA is funded by Congress to conduct these analyses, either in-house or by contract. OTA uses committees to provide expert advice on issues it is evaluating; care is always taken to include representation of the interested public on the committees and to keep the studies free from partisan bias.

The General Accounting Office (GAO) monitors expenditures of congressional appropriations. As part of its overall mission, the GAO conducts studies on the financial issues related to science and technology. As science and technology have become increasingly important functions in the government, the need for expertise in science policy in GAO has grown as well.

The members' constituencies provide a major source of science policy input to Congress as well. Elected officials are the public's representatives in government. Constituents in the respective congressional districts voice their opinions through letters, meetings, and by forming special interest groups. In some cases these activities influence legislation that directly affects overall science and technology policy. Congressional appropriations for research centers, computers, or facilities in a member's district as a result of earmarking are resource allocations that often avoid customary peer review mechanisms.

The National Academy of Sciences was chartered officially by Abraham Lincoln in 1863 to advise the government upon request on scientific and technical matters. Requests quite often are initiated by Congress and carried out under contract from executive agencies. The Academy convenes committees of experts, mostly nongovernmental, to provide information and make recommendations. Thus, the Academy and its associated bodies—the National Academy of Engineering, the Institute of Medicine, and its operating arm, the National Research Council—provide science policy advice to the government upon request.

In 1988 Congress asked the National Academy of Sciences, the National Academy of Engineering, and the Institute of Medicine to provide advice on developing an appropriate institutional framework and information base for conducting cross-program development and review of the nation's R&D programs. The Academy committee identified two overriding questions needing analysis: (1) Is the United States investing adequately for the long term to sustain the enabling science and technology infrastructure? (2) Are priorities among science and technology opportunities decided in a way that best advances the national interest?[7]

The Academy committee's analysis examined all science and technology supported directly by the federal government. This included not only the support of basic and applied research but also related activities such as science and engineering education and the financing and operating of specialized facilities. The analysis considered how public officials perceive, prepare, and review science and technology budgets throughout the federal budgetary cycle. Subsequently, the Academy committee suggested an analytical framework and changes in the federal budget process to aid public officials in decisions about science and technology resources.

The framework proposed by the Academy committee for guiding science and technology budget preparation includes consideration of activities and policy objectives across as well as within agencies. The framework includes analysis of science and technology in four interrelated categories: (1) pertinence to agency mission, (2) investment in the science and technology base, (3) pertinence to national objectives, and (4) new and possibly large science and technology initiatives.[7] Whereas this framework applies to all science and technology, the committee believes it is applicable equally within the health sciences.

Priority Setting Within NIH/ADAMHA

The National Institutes of Health (NIH) and the Alcohol, Drug Abuse, and Mental Health Administration (ADAMHA) are charged with implementing a workable plan for improving human health through basic and applied research. A complex system of interactions between the Executive Branch and Congress helps shape priorities within NIH and ADAMHA. Administrators in the Public Health Service (PHS) and outside advisory groups are responsible for developing and implementing a strategy to achieve these goals.

Office of the Director

The director of NIH, who is a presidential appointee, is primarily responsible for coordinating institute programs and research support divisions along broad policy guidelines. Along with the institute directors, the NIH director must develop NIH's annual budget proposal and defend it before PHS and Congress. In this respect, the director maintains a close liaison with the assistant secretary for health in the Department of Health and Human Services (DHHS), who oversees all activities of the PHS, including budget projections.

The NIH director's support staff consists of three deputy directors and several associate directors. One deputy director shares the overall responsibilities of the director, acting on his behalf. A second deputy director, the deputy director for intramural research, aided by an associate director for intramural affairs and an assistant director for intramural planning, is responsible for intramural research policy in the institutes and divisions. The third deputy director, the deputy director for extramural research and training, along with an associate director for extramural affairs, oversee grant programs supported by the institutes and administered through the Division of Research Grants. The NIH director is aided by the associate director for AIDS research, the associate director for clinical care, the associate director for science policy and legislation, the associate director for administration, the associate director for human genome research, the associate director for communications, and the associate director for international research.

Under the auspices of an associate director, the Office of Science Policy and Legislation performs the central planning for the director and his staff. This office advises the director on external forces that affect NIH's programs and policies. Responsibilities of this office include policy analysis and development, central program planning and evaluation, and interpreting legislation as it pertains to NIH; the office is responsible as well for publishing *NIH Research Plans*, *NIH Evaluation Plans*, *Legislative Highlights and Issues*, and the *NIH Data Book*.

In addition to the guidance provided by the Office of Science Policy and Legislation, the NIH director receives guidance on NIH programs and policies from several advisory committees, some of which are statutory, such as the President's Cancer Panel, the National Arthritis Advisory Board, and the Board of Regents for the National Library of Medicine. Other advisory committees, such as the Director's Advisory Committee, which convenes to advise the director on broad issues affecting NIH research policies, are unofficial advisory groups appointed by the director. The Director's Advisory Committee generally does not provide guidance on the overall NIH research program. Rather, this body of advisors commonly

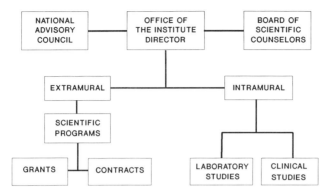

FIGURE 3-2 A typical NIH institute. (Source: U.S. Department of Health and Human Services, Public Health Service. 1988. NIH Peer Review of Research Grant Applications. Bethesda, Md.: National Institutes of Health.)

examines specific cross-cutting issues relating to the research establishment. Several review panels, including the 1976 President's Biomedical Research Panel, that have examined the role of the Director's Advisory Council have recommended that this advisory group be authorized by statute in order to provide a more comprehensive overview of the nation's biomedical research effort.

Institute Planning

A variety of forces formulate and shape institute research strategies. The structure of a typical institute is shown in Figure 3-2. As does the director of NIH, the individual institute directors have staffs for program planning and evaluation, communications, and special functions. Each institute has an extramural component, and most institutes have an intramural component. Extramural scientific programs include grants, contracts, and cooperative agreements, and they are overseen by a scientific director. The intramural program deals with laboratory and clinical studies conducted within NIH facilities.

Institute directors receive advice for institute program planning and direction from various groups of advisors: the Boards of Scientific Counselors and the National Advisory Councils. The Board of Scientific Counselors of each institute advises the institute director on intramural research priorities in those institutes having intramural programs; it is also responsible for assessing the intramural programs as well as periodically reviewing tenured scientists within the institute. Often times special presidentially appointed boards may focus program objectives and research directions such as the National Cancer Advisory Board.

The National Advisory Council of each institute has the authority to define program priorities, primarily by awarding extramural research grants and contracts to investigators in areas it feels are institute priorities. The councils have a broad-based membership of both scientists and lay persons. Generally, they consist of 12 scientists knowledgeable in the field and 6 lay persons as well as ex officio members, such as the institute director and NIH director. The advisory councils do not have scientific support staff nor a budgetary allocation to research issues affecting grants or other extramural awards. Also, there is no official coordination between the Boards of Scientific Counselors overseeing the intramural programs and the National Advisory Councils, which are primarily concerned with the extramural component. Likewise, there is no mechanism for coordinating priorities among the councils of the 13 institutes.

FEDERAL BUDGET PROCESS

Ideally, once all of the advisory mechanisms have provided the government with scientific priorities and goals, a federal budget is developed reflecting this plan. However, because there are so many complexities in formulating the federal budget, the process is never this straightforward. For each fiscal year beginning in October, the President is required by law to submit the budget within 15 days of Congress's convening in the new calendar year, generally by the beginning of February. Since the President's budget is based on agency proposals, the PHS agencies must begin preparing their budget proposals 12 to 15 months in advance of this submission date. Thus, three budgets are being worked on simultaneously: (1) the budget the Executive Branch is developing for 2 years hence, (2) the budget for the next fiscal year on which Congress is having public hearings, and (3) the budget for the current fiscal year that Congress may be revising throughout the year. The following section reviews the federal budget process as well as the specifics for developing the health research budgets for NIH and ADAMHA.

Presidential Budget Development

Agency Budget Requests

Development of the President's budget for health sciences research begins with meetings among agency directors in the DHHS, the Office of the Assistant Secretary for Health (OASH), and the assistant secretary for budget and management. The PHS agencies, including all centers, institutes, and divisions of NIH and ADAMHA, determine their own priorities and desired program levels with the help of outside advisory committees. Several months are devoted to developing program initiatives and evaluating trade-offs for particular funding levels. Subsequently, a formal budget request is submitted to OASH based on estimates for the cost of maintaining current services and supporting additional program objectives. These budgets then are passed on to the DHHS, which evaluates them relative to the health objectives of the department and the nation. Concurrently, the President requires that the OMB, the Council of Economic Advisors, and the Treasury Department make separate projections on federal revenues and obligations.

Office of Management and Budget

The DHHS usually sends its proposed budget to OMB 12 months before the start of the fiscal year (Figure 3-3). OMB examiners review the budget requests of the individual agencies and evaluate program levels, initiatives, and funding requirements. The budget decisions by OMB are influenced by overall administration fiscal policy in the context of the scientific goals proposed by the department. Once OMB completes its review, the budgets are returned to the agencies with OMB's "mark" of the budget targets that the agencies must meet, usually by sometime in December. If a particular agency disagrees with the OMB mark, it can appeal through department channels to the OMB or directly to the President. Once differences are reconciled, a budget is approved formally by the President and submitted to Congress after the first of the year.

In recent years downward negotiations of active research project grant budgets have been specified in the President's budget. For example, the NIH budget request for fiscal year 1989 assumed a 13 percent reduction in the budgets of new research project grant awards and a 10 percent reduction for noncompeting research project grant renewals.

Congressional Budget Process

Three separate but related processes take place in Congress during the development of the federal budget for health sciences research at NIH and ADAMHA. Budgeting, authorization, and appropriation processes are the primary means by which Congress sets its biomedical research priorities. Each of these three processes is dealt with by separate committees in the House and the Senate, with minor variances in committee composition and responsibilities.

Authorizing Committees

Congress must authorize all federal programs prior to the commencement of federal spending; it usually does this for multiyear periods. The Subcommittee on Health and the Environment of the House Committee on Energy and Commerce and the Senate Committee on Labor and Human

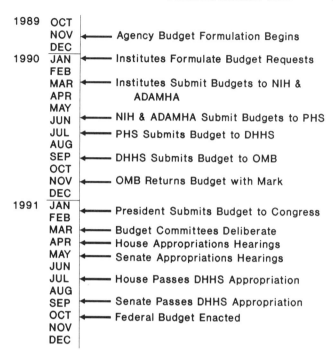

FIGURE 3-3 Time line of federal budget preparation.

Resources initiate authorization bills for research programs in the PHS. This legislation authorizes research activities in the divisions of NIH and ADAMHA as well as specific institutes. Authorization bills also can establish funding levels and time limits on specific programs. This authority to specify program funding levels is the first of many steps Congress takes in shaping the budgets for NIH and ADAMHA. However, the NIH has a continuing authority under section 301 of the Public Health Act. This additional authorizing legislation tends to focus upon specific programs and institutes within the NIH.

Budget Committees

The budget committees of the House and Senate perform an important but nonbinding function in establishing federal budget spending levels. Based on the best estimates from congressional committees overseeing other federal agencies and projections from the Congressional Budget Office (CBO), the budget committees jointly issue a First Concurrent Resolution. This document details government receipts, obligations, public debt, and targets for budget expenditures. To create the final Concurrent

Resolution, a House/Senate conference may be required to reconcile differences between the chambers. The Concurrent Resolution provides key federal guidelines for the appropriations and finance committees. Since the entire congressional budget committee process takes less than 2 months, a detailed analysis of individual federal programs cannot be conducted.

Although the recommendations of the budget committees are nonbinding, the passage of the Deficit Reduction Act has constrained the process somewhat. That is, appropriations committees are prohibited from increasing spending levels for specific line items in the budget beyond small percentages specified by the budget committees. For example, increases in discretionary domestic spending could not exceed $3 billion of the total fiscal year 1989 budget of $38 billion for these programs. For fiscal year 1989, NIH's budget was increased by $500 million—18 percent of the entire allowable increases for all domestic programs.

Appropriations Committees

The recommendations of the budget committees are forwarded to the appropriations committees. In the House and Senate, the 13 subcommittees comprising the appropriations committees each receive allocations for the programs in their purview through the process known as 302b allocations. The House Subcommittee on Labor, Health and Human Services, Education, and Related Agencies is responsible for determining the appropriations for NIH and ADAMHA. In the Senate this same function is performed by the Subcommittee on Labor, Health and Human Services, and Education. One primary difference in the proceedings between the House and Senate is the deferral of training funds by the House. Training is an unauthorized activity, and to decrease procedural time the House defers action. Thus, the Senate determines the federal commitment to training.

The appropriations for the centers, institutes, and divisions of NIH are separate budget line items. The director of NIH and the institute directors are called upon to describe program priorities and provide budget justifications in public hearings during the appropriations process. Therefore, scientific priorities are reflected by fiscal policy in the congressional subcommittees.

The Office of Science Policy and Planning in the Office of the Director of NIH is responsible for responding to congressional activities that pertain to the institutes. On occasion, Congress instructs NIH to undertake specific activities in statutory language of appropriations bills, and NIH must respond with a Legislative Implementation Plan. More commonly, Congress provides NIH with directives through the report language that accompanies the bill. It is possible that three reports can accompany a bill: (1) a Conference Report, (2) a House Report, and (3) a Senate Report.

Of these, the Conference Report is the most binding. However, NIH tries to comply with these directives and negotiates discrepancies between the Senate and House versions when necessary.

Adjusting Allocations

There are mechanisms to adjust the NIH and ADAMHA budgets, up or down, following the enactment of an appropriations bill. The GRH deficit reduction bill automatically cuts federal spending when budget deficits exceed specified annual levels. The NIH and ADAMHA budgets can be revised through supplemental appropriations, transfers, or reprogramming. For example, supplemental appropriations were made to NIH and ADAMHA in 1982, 1983, and 1984 to increase funding for AIDS research. This flexibility in the appropriations process is intended to allow Congress to respond to health emergencies.

The DHHS cannot transfer appropriations among agencies or reprogram funds without congressional approval. Transfers are rare, since in lieu of transfer Congress generally will pass a supplemental appropriations bill. On the other hand, reprogramming is fairly common within agencies, and Congress has mechanisms in place to expedite these requests for redistributing funds between grants, contracts, and intramural programs within the institutes.

Problems Identified by Congress

Through committee reports, Congress identifies its intentions as well as specifies issues needing further attention. For example, the President's budget request for fiscal year 1989 stipulated downward negotiations of 13 and 10 percent for new and continuing grant awards, respectively. However, Congress's report language requested that the NIH director reexamine spending plans to limit downward negotiations while maintaining the number of grants supported above the 1988 levels. The House committee also would not approve a 16.2 percent budget increase to maintain current services for 1989 without an explanation of increasing research costs. Therefore, the committee requested that the inspector general for DHHS review a sampling of extramural awards to determine whether these costs are being well managed.[8]

Congress has been criticized in the past for micromanaging the NIH budget and earmarking funds for special interests, but it is now attempting to limit that activity. The following statement appears in the fiscal year 1989 House Report:

> Beyond expressing its concern about funding for investigator-initiated research grants and policies on downward negotiations, the committee has attempted to minimize its directions to the Institutes regarding the specific allocations related

to individual diseases or research mechanisms. It is the committee's view that these decisions are best made by the scientists and the science managers at NIH based on the quality of the opportunities as they present themselves during the year.[9]

SUMMARY AND CONCLUSIONS

The committee concluded that the process for setting research priorities and developing the federal health budget is very fragmented and deeply embedded in a wide range of political considerations. However, the committee recognized the need for planning among federal agencies to ensure that critical national viewpoints are represented equally well when research priorities concerning use of health sciences research funds are established. Thus, there is a need for a more uniformly accepted priority-setting process that ensures that both scientific and public interests are foremost in the decisions made within the legislative and executive branches of the federal government.

The large federal deficits of the 1980s have put tremendous pressures on all federal budget categories. Passage of the GRH Deficit Reduction Act has intensified budget pressures, forcing all federal agencies to strive to meet current services within federal fiscal guidelines. Agencies with science and technology budgets are subject to these constraints as well but generally have been spared some of the budget cuts other domestic programs have endured.

The federal government will invest more than $71 billion in R&D in fiscal year 1991. Of this, nearly $10 billion will be invested in health sciences R&D. Industry, foundations, and other sources will contribute an equally large amount. In light of these investments as well as recent economic, demographic, and political developments that affect funding and administration of research programs, it will be necessary to develop a process to establish priorities. Effective advisory mechanisms throughout government are necessary. Additionally, the government must draw upon the collective talent of those scientists performing the work within academic institutions.

The committee believes that without better mechanisms for long-range planning, current allocation practices could impede future advances in health sciences research. Continued vitality and progress in health sciences research depend on developing scientific talent and providing adequate laboratories and equipment. The committee believes that more communication among the supporters of health sciences research is needed to maximize the return on the health sciences research investments as well as to restore the balance of support for research projects, training of research personnel, purchasing of instruments, and building or renovation of facilities. The committee concluded that any changes in resource allocation policy should foster synergism in the support of health sciences research and ensure that an optimal research environment is sustained to broaden our knowledge base further. Without careful planning and ongoing oversight, the allocation of resources to meet these needs will be self-defeating.

REFERENCES

1. Ford, G.R. 1988. Science advice to the President. In Science and Technology Advice to the President, Congress, and Judiciary. W.T. Golden, ed. New York: Pergamon Press.
2. Roe, R.A. 1988. Science and technology advice for the President and Congress: The need for a new perspective. In Science and Technology Advice to the President, Congress, and Judiciary. W.T. Golden, ed. New York: Pergamon Press.
3. Buchsbaum, S.J. 1988. On advising the federal government. In Science and Technology Advice to the President, Congress, and Judiciary. W.T. Golden, ed. New York: Pergamon Press.
4. Beckler, D.Z. 1988. Science and technology in presidential policymaking: A new dimension and structure. In Science and Technology Advice to the President, Congress, and Judiciary. W.T. Golden, ed. New York: Pergamon Press.
5. Atkinson, R.C. 1988. Science advice at the cabinet level. In Science and Technology Advice to the President, Congress, and Judiciary. W.T. Golden, ed. New York: Pergamon Press.
6. National Academy of Sciences, National Academy of Engineering, and the Institute of Medicine. 1989. Science and Technology Advice in the White House. Washington, D.C.: National Academy Press.
7. National Academy of Sciences, National Academy of Engineering, and the Institute of Medicine. 1989. Federal Science and Technology Budget Priorities: New Perspectives and Procedures. Washington D.C.: National Academy Press.
8. U.S. Department of Health and Human Services; Office of the Inspector General. 1989. Survey on the Cost of Research at Colleges and Universities. Publication No. A-12-89-00128. Washington, D.C.
9. U.S. House of Representatives. 1989. Report of the House of Representatives Appropriations Subcommittee for the Departments of Labor, Health and Human Services, and Education, and Related Agencies Appropriations Bill, 1989. Report No. 100-689. Washington, D.C.

4
Supporting Research Through
NIH and ADAMHA

As previously discussed, nearly half of all financial support for health sciences research comes from federal sources (see Chapter 2). Of this, about 78 percent is disbursed through the National Institutes of Health (NIH) and the Alcohol, Drug Abuse, and Mental Health Administration (ADAMHA).

The NIH has become a world-renowned and highly respected biomedical research organization with a mission to uncover new knowledge that will lead to better health for everyone.[1] Currently, NIH consists of 13 categorical institutes, 2 support divisions, 4 specialized centers, the Clinical Center, the Fogarty International Center, and the National Library of Medicine, all located primarily on a 300-acre tract in Bethesda, Maryland (Figure 4-1).

Unlike some foreign governmental support for medical research, only a small proportion of federally sponsored biomedical research actually is conducted in U.S. federal laboratories. Nearly 80 percent of the NIH budget is allocated to research and training at universities and other research institutions, both in the United States and abroad.[2] Most of these funds are allocated through peer review processes that include the views of scientists and others throughout the country. Therefore, the NIH is a decentralized organization with scientific priorities determined by individual investigators, Congress, and other interested parties.

The ADAMHA is responsible for advancing scientific knowledge to improve the understanding, prevention, and treatment of alcohol abuse and alcoholism, drug abuse, and mental health disorders.[3] ADAMHA is

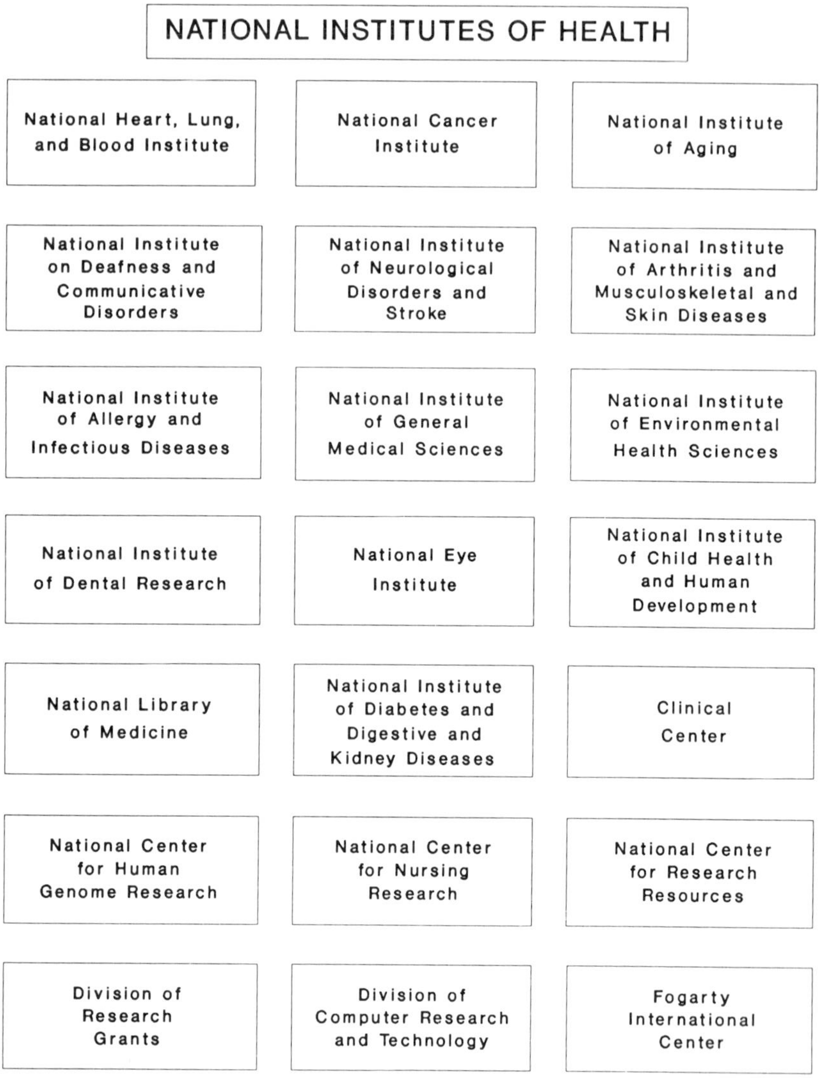

FIGURE 4-1   The institutes, centers, and divisions of the National Institutes of Health.

composed of three separate institutes: the National Institute on Alcohol Abuse and Alcoholism, the National Institute on Drug Abuse, and the National Institute of Mental Health (Figure 4-2). In addition to conducting and supporting biomedical and behavioral research and research training, ADAMHA is responsible for demonstrations, clinical training, treatment, prevention, and public information activities on public health problems

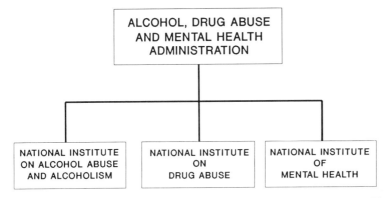

FIGURE 4-2   The research institutes of the Alcohol, Drug Abuse, and Mental Health Administration.

related to its mission. The peer review process and programs for research and training support are in most ways identical to NIH.

Federal funding programs for supporting research and research training outside of federal laboratories are primarily grants, cooperative agreements (financial assistance awards), and contracts (acquisition awards). At NIH and ADAMHA these are referred to collectively as "extramural" programs and fall into five major categories: research grants, research and development (R&D) contracts, research training awards, cooperative agreements, and construction authority (NIH only). R&D grants have been and continue to be the cornerstone of NIH and ADAMHA extramural support for health research since the expansion of the NIH extramural programs began in the mid 1940s.

ALLOCATIONS FOR NIH AND ADAMHA

The policy change following World War II to advance basic knowledge by supporting civilian R&D in academic institutions stimulated steady increases in the NIH budget (Figure 2-6). This growth has resulted because of the emphasis society has chosen to give to health research and because of the subsequent legislation that created numerous new institutes and expanded the extramural programs of NIH. The most rapid budget growth occurred between 1955 and 1965—a period of expansion. From the late 1960s to 1980, budget growth leveled off and may be referred to as steady state. During the 1980s, congressional appropriations to NIH increased an average of 10 percent per year, resulting in a 2 percent per annum real growth in the NIH budget (Figure 4-3).[1] However, much of the increases of the past few years can be attributed to the growth in funding for AIDS research.

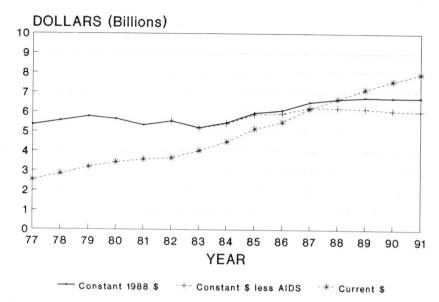

FIGURE 4-3 NIH appropriations with and without allocations for AIDS research from 1977 to 1991. (Appendix Table A-7) Note: Constant dollar calculations are made using the BRDPI deflator.

Allocations among NIH extramural and intramural programs and program management have not changed significantly since the late 1970s (Figure 4-4). Extramural programs account for nearly 80 percent of the NIH budget. The intramural program has remained at 10 to 12 percent of the budget over the same period. Program management, which includes the Office of the Director, Division of Research Grants, and the National Library of Medicine, has been receiving successively smaller percentages of the NIH budget, falling to 7 percent in 1989 from nearly 10 percent in 1977.

Although appropriations for ADAMHA grew and paralleled those of NIH throughout the 1970s, the agency budget was cut in the early 1980s. Cuts in social sciences research and nonresearch community programs, recommended by the Reagan administration and enacted by Congress in the early 1980s, drastically reduced total ADAMHA appropriations.[4] Only recently have appropriations for ADAMHA surpassed the 1979 level. The President's budget proposal for fiscal year 1991 requests more than $2.8 billion for ADAMHA (Figure 4-5).[5]

Community programs have been and continue to be the largest portion of the ADAMHA budget, ranging from 53 to 61 percent of the ADAMHA budget over the past 10 years (Figure 4-6). Obligations for research grew from 17 percent to 33 percent of the budget in the same period. When measured in constant 1988 dollars, there has been an average annual growth of 3.5 percent in this part of the budget since 1977 (Figures 4-5 and 4-6). However, there have been wide annual variances in research support, ranging from a 12 percent cut in 1981 to an 18 percent increase in 1987.[5] Recently, the rapid growth in ADAMHA's research budget reflects the government's priority for combating drug abuse through basic research.

Since these two agencies are the primary federal sponsors of health sciences research, this chapter examines their research support programs. Although the support programs for research projects cannot be separated easily from training and facilities (Chapters 5 and 6), the committee tried to isolate them for the purposes of this review. To this end, this chapter explores the policies that have affected the levels of support as well as the number and types of research project support programs available from NIH and ADAMHA. The chapter also examines the characteristics and trends of the scientists performing research sponsored by NIH and ADAMHA.

NIH DIRECT OPERATIONS

Appropriations for research support divisions, extramural grant management, and for the National Library of Medicine (NLM) have not kept pace with inflation. In constant 1988 dollars, funding for program support

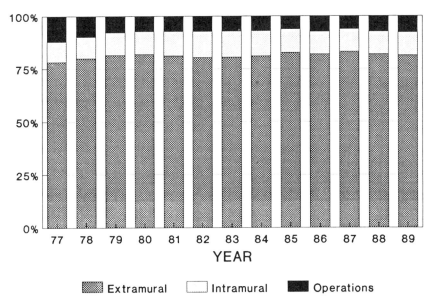

FIGURE 4-4   Allocation of NIH budget from 1977 to 1989. (Appendix Table A-8)

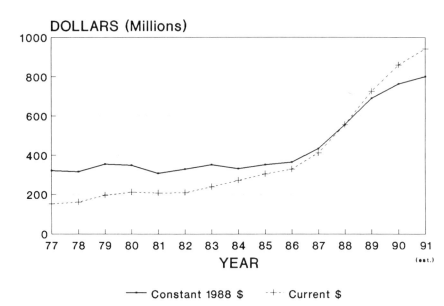

FIGURE 4-5   ADAMHA research allocations from 1977 to 1990. (Appendix Table A-9)

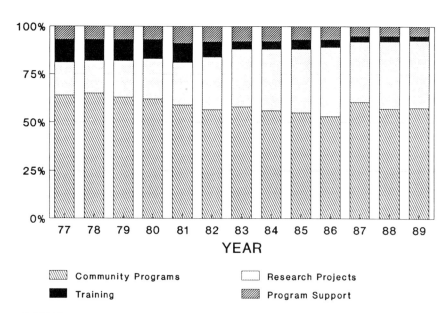

FIGURE 4-6   Allocation of ADAMHA budget from 1977 to 1989. (Appendix A-10)

and management has declined by 30 percent. Likewise, the NLM budget has declined by 17 percent. Funding for the Office of the Director has remained fairly constant at 0.6 to 0.7 percent of the entire NIH budget.

Intramural Research

The largest portion of NIH funds for direct activities is allocated to the intramural research programs in the 13 institutes. Intramural program activities include basic research, clinical research, scientist training, communication of scientific findings, development of policies on biomedical research priorities, and translation of research findings into more effective medical care.[6] Although none of these functions is unique to the intramural program, the intramural program is distinct in the federal portfolio of support for health research. The key features of the intramural program include freedom from competitive grant procedures; unique research resources, including the Warren Grant Magnuson Clinical Center; and research related directly to the individual institute missions.

Whereas the intramural programs were allocated sizeable portions of the NIH budget during the early postwar expansion, allocations for the intramural program were stable throughout the 1980s at 10 to 12 percent of the total NIH budget (Figure 4-4). Some institutes, such as the National Cancer Institute (NCI) and the National Institute of Environmental Health Sciences (NIEHS), invest heavily in their intramural programs, whereas others, such as the National Institute of General Medical Sciences (NIGMS), have no significant intramural programs. In constant dollars, funding for the intramural programs has increased from $521 million in 1977 to $757 million in 1990 (Figure 4-7). This reflects a 2 percent per year real growth in the intramural budget that parallels the overall growth in the NIH budget over the same period.[6]

During the 1980s, there was speculation that the intramural research program was not performing at the level of quality characteristic of it in the past. Whereas the NIH campus served as a primary training ground for health scientists in the 1950s and 1960s, there were signs in the 1980s that the NIH was beginning to have difficulty attracting and retaining outstanding basic scientists and clinical investigators. These deficiencies have been attributed to relatively low government salary scales, noncompetitive fringe benefits, and the other bureaucratic constraints of working in a federal agency.

In response to these concerns and to the suggestion that the intramural program could benefit by shifting to the private sector, the Institute of Medicine (IOM) conducted an in-depth review of the program in 1988.[6] The IOM study committee concluded that the intramural program has

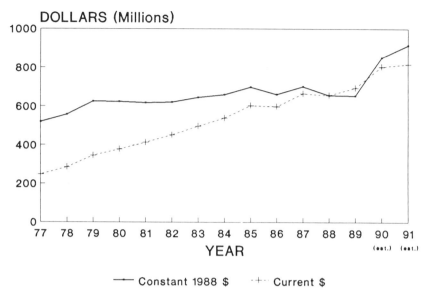

FIGURE 4-7   NIH obligations for intramural research from 1977 to 1991. (Appendix A-8)

previously made and continues to make valuable contributions to understanding basic biological and disease processes. Despite NIH's difficulties in coordinating activities across institutes effectively and in responding efficiently to new challenges or crises, the IOM study committee also concluded that the federated organizational structure of NIH has helped meet the nation's biomedical research needs. In order to maintain the intramural program's excellence and credibility and to improve deficient areas, the study committee recommended some changes in NIH administration as well as in the scope of responsibilities of scientific administrators directing the intramural programs.

The recommendations of the Institute's NIH intramural study committee were as follows:

• To increase administrative efficiency, the committee recommended that the Secretary of Health and Human Services delegate to the director of NIH the authority to make decisions on administrative matters without being subject to review by the Office of the Assistant Secretary for Health.

• To increase NIH's ability to respond more effectively to emerging issues, new opportunities, and crises not confined to any single institute, the committee recommended that Congress annually appropriate a $25 million director's fund to be used to address these issues.

• To enhance the quality of the intramural program, the committee recommended that a formal review panel be established to evaluate each institute's scientific directors and intramural programs quadrennially.

• To be competitive, the committee believes that NIH has to exercise greater flexibility in the labor market and therefore recommended that Congress authorize NIH to develop and implement a demonstration project to overcome current staffing deficiencies.

• To attract high-level scientists from outside government service, the committee recommended that Congress charter a foundation to permit private support for endowing 10 chairs for distinguished investigators.

• To attract junior-level investigators, the committee recommended that Congress authorize and appropriate funds to create an NIH Scholars Program in which outstanding young investigators at the assistant professor level are appointed on a competitive basis to independent, nontenured positions in the intramural program.

This committee concurs with the intramural study committee that these measures will enhance the intramural program as the flagship of U.S. biomedical research.

NIH Extramural Programs: R&D Grants

R&D grants, particularly investigator-initiated research project grants (R01), continue to be the cornerstone of the NIH extramural program (Table 4-1 and Figure 4-4). As growth in the NIH budget slowed during the 1970s, competition for grants intensified, and the number of new and competing renewal grants awarded by NIH fluctuated annually. Through the 1970s the number of proposals funded ranged from as few as 3,500 in 1976 to 5,900 in 1979 (Figure 4-8); this number did not follow any particular pattern but depended on the cumulative grant portfolio and funds available in any particular institute.

Initially, the 1976 Report of the President's Biomedical Research Panel brought to light the issue of fluctuating numbers of NIH and ADAMHA research project grant proposals being funded annually.[7] By the end of 1970s, these fluctuations had increased and had caused even deeper notions of instability in the support of biomedical research. The 1979 and 1980 reports by the Health and Human Services (HHS) Steering Committee for the Development of a Health Research Strategy reexamined these concerns about the future of federal support for new as well as ongoing health research in light of impending federal budget constraints. These reports called for 5-year plans and evaluative procedures to be established for all of the health-related agencies in HHS.[8,9] The 1979 Steering Committee report also emphasized the need to stabilize the science base by making investigator-initiated research projects the first priority in the NIH and ADAMHA research budgets. As a result, Congress and the Executive

TABLE 4-1 NIH Research Grants* by Kind and Type, 1988 (dollars in thousands)

Kind of Grant and Code	Number	Amount
Total	25,754	$4,727,320
Research projects	20,867	3,764,791
Traditional (R01)	16,871	2,564,198
Research program projects (P01)	770	634,809
New investigator research (R23)	260	11,920
SBIR (R43, R44)	460	54,334
MERIT awards (R37)	596	140,829
Outstanding investigator (R35)	74	46,985
FIRST awards (R29)	1,227	108,253
Other (R22, U01, P42)	609	203,463
Research centers	621	573,578
Specialized (P50)	192	164,531
Core grants (P30)	176	165,586
General clinical (M01)	78	102,159
Comprehensive (P60)	36	47,920
Biotechnology resource (P41, U41)	70	36,697
Primate research center (P51)	7	33,300
Animal resource (P40, U40)	42	12,064
RCMIs (G12)	19	11,010
Other (P20)	1	310
Other research	4,266	388,952
Biomedical research support & development (S03, S07, S10)	1,110	90,918
RCPAs (K)	1,443	94,586
Cooperative clinical (R10, U10)	331	80,268
Minority biomedical support (S06, S11, S14)	102	83,407
Other	1,280	83,407

*Represents awards, not obligations.

SOURCE: U.S. Department of Health and Human Services. 1989. NIH Data Book 1989. National Institutes of Health Publication No. 90-1261. Bethesda, Md.

Branch agreed on a policy that specified the minimum number of new and competing grants NIH and ADAMHA would be required to fund each year—"stabilization policy."

The 1979 Steering Committee report suggested that the minimum number of competitive research grant awards for fiscal year 1981 be 5,000 for NIH and 569 for ADAMHA.[4] From 1981 to 1988 increasing minimum numbers of new and competing research grants to be awarded were specified in either report or statutory language accompanying congressional appropriations bills. Whereas the initial NIH base was established at 5,000, the administration requested funding for only 284 awards for ADAMHA in 1981—only half the recommended level. However, this was modified upward by Congress to 345. Throughout the 1980s, the number of new and competing proposals to be funded became an integral part of the federal budget ritual. By 1987 grant awards exceeded 6,400 for NIH and ADAMHA awarded nearly 600. In 1988, the last year of stabilization, NIH funded 6,200 grant awards.

Despite added appropriations from congressional committees, the funds available were never adequate to fund fully the agreed upon number of awards. In order to comply, NIH and ADAMHA were forced into a policy of reducing ongoing research commitments (continuing awards for already approved and funded grants) as well as the amounts paid to new and competing awards in what is commonly referred to as "downward negotiation"—a recent practice for reconciling NIH and ADAMHA research grant commitments to annual appropriations by making across-the-board reductions in all grant awards. Downward negotiation is a euphemism, for little if any negotiation actually occurs between the scientist and NIH or ADAMHA. Rather, these decisions concerning the overall proportions of the previously committed funds to be withheld in order to fund the required annual level of new and competing awards are made between the NIH or ADAMHA and the Office of Management and Budget (OMB). Actually, downward negotiations are administrative budget cuts in the grant awards. This policy has placed additional burdens on scientists,

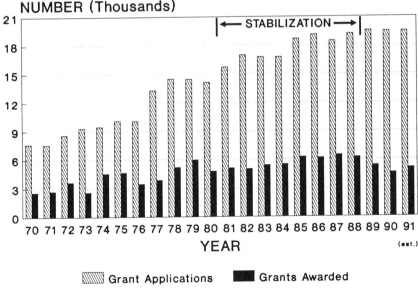

FIGURE 4-8 Number of grant applications submitted to NIH and the number of grants awarded from 1970 to 1991. (Appendix A-11)

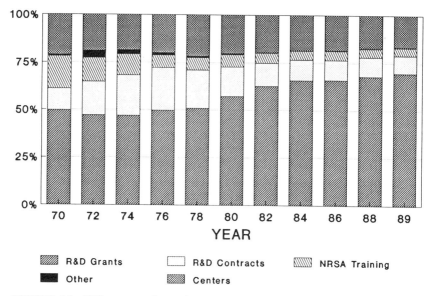

FIGURE 4-9 NIH extramural awards as a percent of extramural activity from 1970 to 1989. (Appendix A-12)

for they are now expected to perform the research proposed with less than the recommended amount of funding.

The committee concluded that the stabilization policy prevented erosion of the nation's scientific base by maintaining minimum annual numbers of investigator-initiated research grants. Research project grants increased from 51 percent of the total NIH extramural budget in 1978 to 67 percent in 1989 (Figure 4-9). Funding for these grew from $2.5 billion in 1977 to $3.9 billion by 1989 when measured in constant 1988 dollars (Figure 4-10). This is the only portion of the NIH extramural budget that has grown in constant dollars over the past decade.

As competition for funding intensified throughout the 1980s, the number of grant applications with very high-priority scores increased. Nevertheless, despite high-priority scores, any given ongoing project faced termination if its score in competitive renewal fell just below the pay line. With interrupted funding, individual scientists felt they would be forced to reduce staff below critical levels so that although amended applications might ultimately restore funding to the program, the research team may by then have already been disbanded. As a consequence of these fears, multiple grant applications, with renewals in alternate years, were seen by many scientists as a means to provide continuity of funding for their research programs.

While NIH and ADAMHA were increasing the numbers of new and

competing awards through the stabilization policy, the research community felt that the average 3-year award period for traditional research project grants (R01) was too short. Three-year awards do not allow for long-term research program planning nor, in many cases, sufficient time to achieve research goals. Additionally, these shorter-duration awards required more frequent renewals and therefore placed too much emphasis on grant writing and administrative details.

Beginning in 1986, NIH and ADAMHA instituted a policy to increase the length of grant awards gradually. One intended result of increasing award periods was to provide more stability in research activities and scientists' careers and, possibly, to discourage the number of multiple grant applications by individual investigators. Additionally, longer award periods were viewed as a means to reduce the administrative workload for NIH and ADAMHA study sections by reducing the number of competitive renewal applications processed each year.

Although increasing grant duration has a stabilizing effect on research careers, it also obligates NIH and ADAMHA appropriations further into the future. This policy of lengthening award periods, coupled with the phenomenon of increasing average award size, reduces the funds available for meeting annual targets of new and competing grant awards. In fact, obligations for noncompeting continuations have grown from 67-68 percent

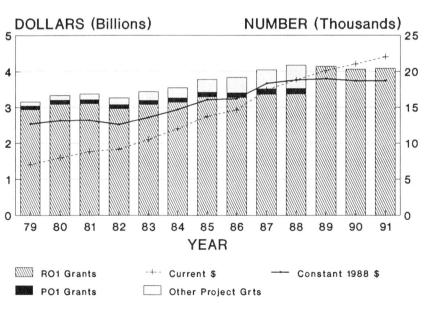

FIGURE 4-10   NIH allocations for research project grants and number supported from 1979 to 1991. (Appendix A-13)

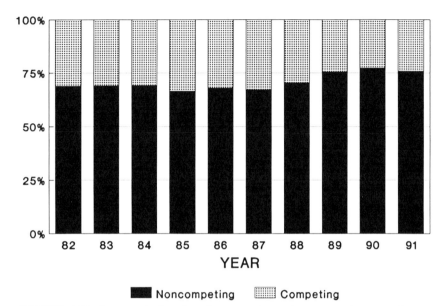

■ Noncompeting   ▦ Competing

FIGURE 4-11 Percent of allocations for competing and noncompeting research grant awards from 1982 to 1991. (Source: National Institutes of Health, Office of Science Policy and Legislation).

of the NIH extramural research budget in the mid 1980s to more than 76 percent in 1990 (Figure 4-11). Although this is a small percentage shift, these growing obligations to noncompeting awards represent about $350 million that is not available for funding new and competing renewal grant applications. As a result, NIH awarded only about 5,400 new and competing awards in 1989; this figure is expected to drop further to nearly 4,600 in 1990.[10]

The total number of research project grants sponsored by NIH grew from 15,500 to 20,867 between 1977 and 1988. In 1989, however, the total number of grants dropped to 20,681, and the number is expected to drop yet even further in 1990 to 20,316. A small gain is expected in the proposed 1991 budget to 20,439. Similarly, the ADAMHA research grant portfolio grew from 1,250 to more than 1,900 over the same period. As a result of the growth of research project grants, other extramural categories have received less and less of the total extramural budget (Figure 4-9).[11]

SETTING PROGRAM PRIORITIES THROUGH PEER REVIEW

Priority Scores

Peer review of competitive proposals forms the core of the NIH/ADAMHA extramural grants program.[12] The process generally takes a

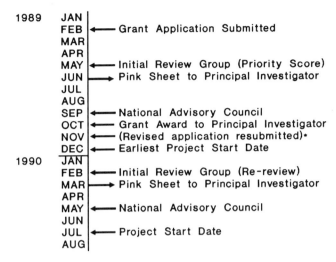

```
1989    JAN
        FEB  ◄──── Grant  Application  Submitted
        MAR
        APR
        MAY  ◄──── Initial  Review  Group  (Priority  Score)
        JUN  ───►  Pink  Sheet  to  Principal  Investigator
        JUL
        AUG
        SEP  ◄──── National  Advisory  Council
        OCT  ◄──── Grant  Award  to  Principal  Investigator
        NOV  ◄──── (Revised  application  resubmitted)•
        DEC  ◄──── Earliest  Project  Start  Date
1990    JAN
        FEB  ◄──── Initial  Review  Group  (Re-review)
        MAR  ───►  Pink  Sheet  to  Principal  Investigator
        APR
        MAY  ◄──── National  Advisory  Council
        JUN
        JUL  ◄──── Project  Start  Date
        AUG
```

FIGURE 4-12 Application time line for new R01 research grant and resubmission of revised application.

minimum of 9 months, from application deadline to final award, for new investigator-initiated grant applications (Figure 4-12). The peer review process for research project grant applications is based on two sequential levels of review; the first level is review by a select group of scientist peers serving on the so-called study sections, and the second level is a review (consisting of approval or disapproval) by the National Advisory Council for the respective NIH institute, center, or division (Figure 4-13).[13]

Applications for research project grants are submitted to NIH's Division of Research Grants (DRG), which serves as the central receiving point for applications submitted to NIH and ADAMHA. The DRG reviews each application for relevance to the overall mission of the Public Health Service (PHS) agencies and assigns the application to the most appropriate Initial Review Group (IRG), also known as study section (program project grant applications are assigned directly to IRGs within the respective institute). These IRGs perform the first level of scientific peer review, during which a priority score is assigned to the research proposal.

The DRG has 71 chartered IRGs, with 12 to 20 members each. In certain cases special study sections or ad hoc groups are convened to review applications not falling into the purview of any particular study section. The study sections are grouped according to scientific disciplines and not by institute. Therefore, several study sections may refer grants to a single institute, or a study section may refer grant applications to different institutes.

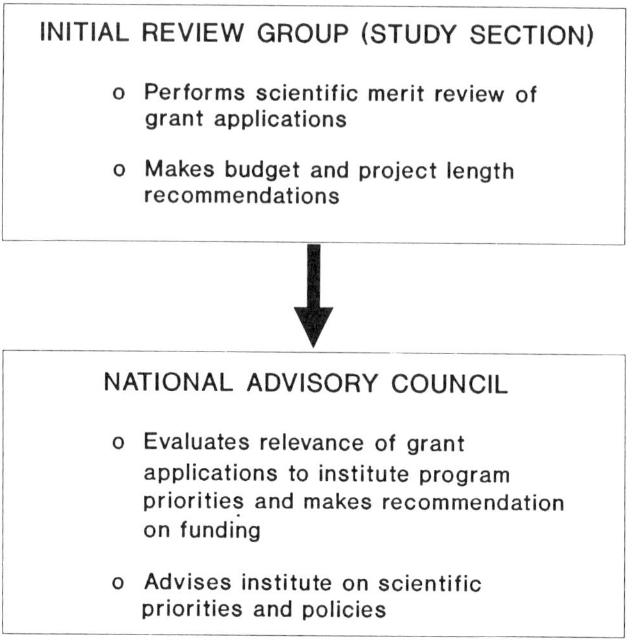

INITIAL REVIEW GROUP (STUDY SECTION)

o Performs scientific merit review of
   grant applications

o Makes budget and project length
   recommendations

NATIONAL ADVISORY COUNCIL

o Evaluates relevance of grant
   applications to institute program
   priorities and makes recommendation
   on funding

o Advises institute on scientific
   priorities and policies

FIGURE 4-13 Schematic diagram of the dual review system used for evaluating and awarding NIH and ADAMHA research grants. (Source: Modified from U.S. Department of Health and Human Services, Public Health Service. 1988. NIH Peer Review of Research Grant Applications. Bethesda, Md.: National Institutes of Health.)

Study sections are composed mainly of nonfederal scientists representing a wide range of specialties; these sections evaluate applications for scientific and technical merit. In most cases investigators have to demonstrate through preliminary studies that the proposed experiments can be completed if funds are awarded. Previous accomplishments by the investigator, including publications, are considered during proposal review. If an investigator does not receive an award with an initial application, an amended or revised proposal can be resubmitted for another grant review cycle. Thus, the application-to-award period can be 18 months or longer (Figure 4-12).

Each proposal receives an in-depth reading from at least two study section members (primary and secondary reviewers) and limited review by the remaining members of the section. When the study section meets, the two reviewers discuss the proposal's scientific merit with their colleagues, and all reviewers in the section then vote on whether to approve or disapprove the application. If approved, all members of the review panel assign a priority score to the proposal; these scores range from 1.0 to 5.0

in tenths of a point, and lower scores indicate a higher priority. Individual scores are averaged and then converted into a scale ranging from 100 to 500 by the executive secretary of the study section. The raw priority score and the review panel comments are compiled into a critique (pink sheet) and sent to the applicant.

A surge in the number of NIH grant applications in recent years has led to concern that certain study sections may be overloaded with proposals to review, although *DRG Peer Review Trends* (1986) indicates that, on average, study sections now handle fewer applications per member than in 1981.[13] However, averages may be misleading, because workloads vary and depend on subject matter and number of proposals received. Study sections also tend to be focused highly on specific research disciplines, and the committee believes that they may be ill-equipped to deal with the multidisciplinary nature of many research questions. Nonetheless, there have been concomitant increases in the number of special study sections and ad hoc groups to offset the increasing number of applications and changes in research directions.

Award Rates

The percent of NIH grant proposals receiving scores of 100 to 150 has more than doubled since 1978, with a concomitant drop in those receiving scores above 300 (Figure 4-14).[11] Also, the approval rate for grant proposals has increased from 70 percent in the mid 1970s to nearly 95 percent in 1989 (Figure 4-15). The improved scores and the increasing approval rates may be the result of several factors including the following: (1) improved grant writing skills as trainees spend longer periods of time in training programs, (2) new and better tools for conducting health research, (3) more amended or resubmitted proposals that receive better scores on the second or third attempt, and (4) behavioral changes by reviewers who know that even excellent proposals will not be funded if they are not ranked in the very top percentiles.

Previously, grant awards were made by order of the priority ranking assigned by the study sections and approved by the advisory councils. However, a recent change to awarding grants by percentile rank has been enacted because of variances among the rankings of the various study sections. In the past, for example, two study sections may have submitted excellent grant proposals to a particular institute. However, because one study section may have ranked good proposals lower overall, the possibility existed that none of its reviewed grants would be funded. By contrast, study sections that ranked proposals higher had a better chance of being awarded in a system that relied on raw priority scores.

The new system arranges the raw priority scores from the present

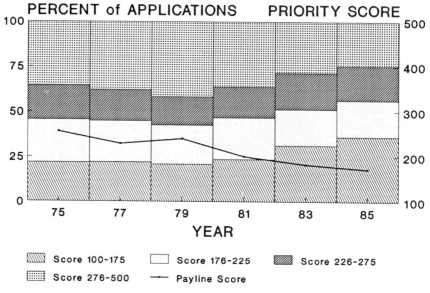

FIGURE 4-14 Distribution of priority scores for R01 research grant applications from 1975 to 1985.[11]

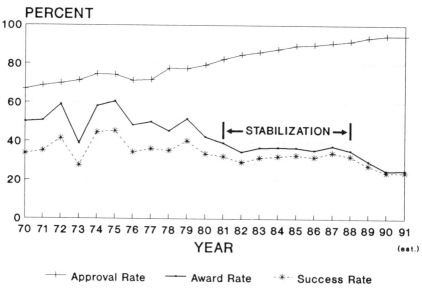

FIGURE 4-15 Approval, award, and success rates for NIH research project grant applications from 1970 to 1991. (Appendix Table A-11)

review cycle and the two previous review cycles of a study section into percentiles. Awards by the institutes are then made by determining a percentile cut-off point. Thus, percentiling normalizes the priority scores of each study section, thereby reducing the variances among the various review panels. However, this change has led to some confusion in translating percentile cut-off points into award rates.

As a result of the increasing priority scores, the average pay line scores—the cut-off point for funding—dropped from more than 200 in the 1970s to less than 150 in 1989 (Figure 4-14). Simultaneously, a decreasing proportion of these applications are awarded funding (Figure 4-15).[11] Thus, the average NIH award rate, the percent of approved applications funded, declined from 60 percent in 1975 to 29 percent for 1989, and it is expected to drop below 25 percent in 1990 (Figure 4-15). However, there are large variances among the institutes—from 30 percent in the National Institute of Arthritis, Musculoskeletal, and Skin Diseases to 50 percent in the National Eye Institute for 1988. The dramatic decline in the overall award rate is moderated somewhat when the success rate, the percentage of total applications funded, is considered. Success rates at NIH have hovered between 35 and 40 percent over this same time period. Yet, as the approval rate edges closer to 100 percent, this discrepancy between award and success rates disappears.[11]

ADAMHA also has experienced increases in the priority scores in its proposal review system, albeit not to the extent of NIH. ADAMHA also experienced an increase in annual grant applications from about 1,800 in 1978 to 2,750 in 1988. The average award rate for research project grants has not declined as rapidly as that of NIH, hovering between 40 and 50 percent since the late 1970s.[4,5] Although this is much higher than NIH, a smaller proportion of ADAMHA grant applications are approved by the peer review panels. When the success rates are considered, the average annual success rates for ADAMHA grant applications have not exceeded the 28 percent level attained in 1979.

An NIH peer review committee was formed in 1987 to examine the current review process.[14] Among the major conclusions and recommendations from that review were the following: (1) innovative or multidisciplinary research should be reemphasized and enhanced by small grant mechanisms, (2) the number of pages in the experimental design and methods section of the grant application should be limited in order to ease the burden on the review process, (3) grant application submission via computer diskettes and electronic mail could accelerate the review process, and (4) applicants should be able to suggest several study sections to simplify the review process and use peer review resources more efficiently. Responding to these recommendations, in 1987 NIH implemented a 20-page limitation (with no more than 10 appendices) on grant applications. Also, NIH currently has a trial project under way involving electronic submissions of grant proposals in hopes of shortening the 9-month grant cycle. An exception to the normal review period is the accelerated proposal review employed for AIDS-related research grants.

In the spring of 1988, an experiment forcing reviewers to use increments of 0.5 rather than 0.1 when assigning priority scores did not affect the priority score distribution significantly. Another suggested potential solution, that of increasing the number of readers for each proposal, has been met with strong opposition because of an anticipated increased workload on the study section members.[17] However, it was the committee's opinion that having more readers would include more scientific judgment in the final priority score.

National Advisory Councils

Once a priority score has been assigned, those proposals pertinent to a particular institute's mission are sent to a second review panel—the National Advisory Council. Each institute has a council that defines its program priorities and officially makes awards to investigators. Whereas the study sections evaluate proposals for their scientific merit, the councils concentrate more on a proposal's importance in terms of the institute's goals. The councils also advise the director and program managers on institute matters concerning overall program priorities and policies.

The councils have a broad-based membership of scientific, professional, and public sector leaders with expertise and interest in the institute's program areas. Generally, the councils consist of 12 scientists knowledgeable in the field and 6 volunteers from the nonscience community with a demonstrated interest in the discipline.[15] The councils do not have scientific support staff, nor do they have a budgetary allocation to investigate research issues affecting grants or other extramural awards. As a result, the councils generally approve a slate of grants proposed by program staff. Following council action, the grant proposals are returned to the DRG, which is responsible for administering the grant awards. However, decisions are made by the councils regarding proposals near the cut-off point and proposals submitted in response to requests to meet institute initiatives.

In most institutes there is no official coordination between the Board of Scientific Counselors for the intramural program and the National Advisory Council, who oversees the extramural component.* Likewise, there is no

---

*NCI's intramural program has more direct control over the extramural program than do the other institutes.

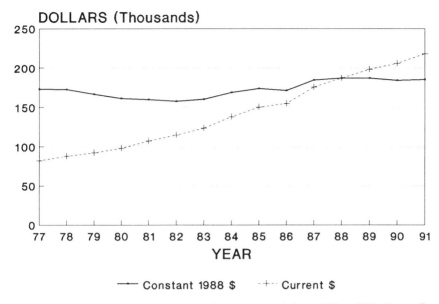

DOLLARS (Thousands)

——— Constant 1988 $ ⁺⁻ Current $

FIGURE 4-16   Average size of research project grant awards from 1977 to 1991. (Appendix Table A-14)

mechanism for coordinating priorities among the councils of the 13 separate institutes, which can create inconsistencies in the overall NIH program.

Trends in Grant Size

The average size of NIH research project grant (RPG) awards has grown from $82,200 per year in 1977 to $198,100 per year in 1990 (direct and indirect costs included) (Figure 4-16). In 1988 constant dollars, the true increase in research project grant size has been from $167,000 to $177,000, reflecting a 5 percent increase. However, the growth rates of different types of research grants vary widely. Between 1977 and 1988 the average size of R01 grants grew from $67,400 to $155,000. Adjusting for inflation this reflects an 11 percent growth, or about one percent per year. By contrast, the average size of program project grants declined by nearly 26 percent in real terms over the same period. Since its inception in 1983, Small Business Innovation Research grants nearly doubled in real terms by 1988, although they account for a small portion of the extramural research budget.

Several factors may have contributed to these award increases, the most significant being personnel costs. Personnel costs, which account for 63 to 72 percent of the research project grant direct costs, rose throughout the award period. The General Accounting Office (GAO) has speculated that higher wages, more experienced personnel, increased numbers of personnel through project expansion, or less voluntary help may account for this increase.[16] The cost of new and more sophisticated equipment also may have added to the increasing grant awards size. However, this committee noted that the percent of research project awards allocated for permanent laboratory equipment dropped from nearly 12 percent in 1966 to less than 4 percent by 1989.[17]

Several other factors may directly affect the size of research project grants including the following: the Biomedical Research and Development Price Index (BRDPI) adjustment for inflation used by NIH; the mix of new, competing renewal, and continuation grants funded in a particular year; indirect cost recovery; increasing complexity of research; increasing regulations on animal use; and increasing use of human subjects.

RESEARCH SCIENTIST TRENDS

Applicant Trends

The percentage of applicants funded on their first attempt varied in the 1970s: from about 24 percent in 1973 to more than 40 percent in 1975. However, in the 1980s the rate stabilized at just under 30 percent. Thus, about half of all applicants will receive a grant award if they apply persistently every year. This is demonstrated in Figure 4-17 which shows the percent of applicants for NIH research projects grant support by year of initial applications from fiscal year 1970 through 1986. This cohort analysis of first-time applicants was limited to traditional research project (R01), new investigator research award (R23), and First Independent Research Support and Transition (FIRST) award (R29) applications.[11]

As shown in Figure 4-8, the number of NIH grant applications has increased considerably in recent years; Ph.D. applicants largely account for this growth. This is particularly true for first-time applicants of traditional research grants (R01) (Figure 4-18). The number of first-time Ph.D. applicants has grown from 1,200 in 1965 to nearly 2,000 in 1985. Fifty-four percent of the first-time R01 applicants in 1965 had a Ph.D. degree compared to 80 percent in 1985.

Over the same period, the number of first-time R01 applicants with M.D. degrees has declined 15 percent, from 950 in 1965 to 800 in 1985. This translates into 28 percent of the first-time applicant pool having an M.D. degree in 1985, compared to 41 percent in 1965. Approximately 100 M.D./Ph.D.s are first-time applicants for NIH funding each year, which also translates into a smaller percentage of the total first-time applicant pool. First-time M.D./Ph.D. and Ph.D. applicants have a slightly higher

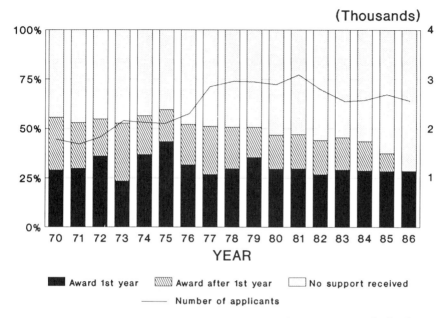

FIGURE 4-17 Percent of applicants for NIH research project grant support by fiscal year of first application from 1970 to 1986.[11]

approval rate than M.D. applicants, but the approval rate trends for all three subgroups are parallel. The trends of first-time R01 recipients parallels that of the first-time applicants (Figure 4-19).

Investigator Turnover

As NIH funds more new and competing awards, it supports more principal investigators. However, the half-life of NIH support for investigators, a measure of time in which one-half of the grant recipients leave the NIH-supported system, has declined continuously since the 1940s. From 1945 to 1954, the median survival time for an investigator in the system ranged from 13 to 21 years. By 1960 the half-life of investigators had dropped to less than 7 years, and it currently stands at less than 6 years.[18] Thus, it appears that as entry rates go up, median survival time goes down as investigators have more difficulty with their competing renewal applications.

Many factors contribute to the higher turnover rate of principal investigators. Much discussion and analysis have focused on award periods. Although the average length of R01s has increased to nearly 4 years since 1977 (Figure 4-20), it has been suggested that young investigators need more than the usual 3-year award to set up and become productive. NIH

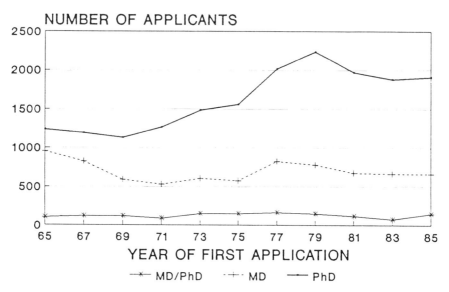

FIGURE 4-18 First-time R01 grant applicants by degree from 1965 to 1985. (Source: NIH Deputy Director for Extramural Research, and Division of Research Grants)

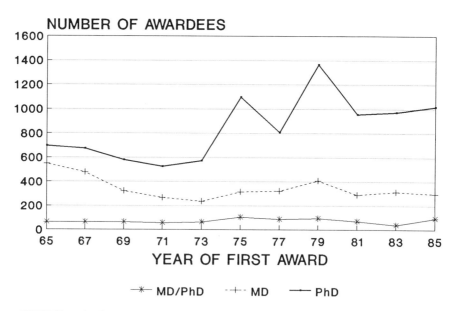

FIGURE 4-19 First-time R01 grant recipients by degree from 1965 to 1985. (Source: NIH Deputy Director for Extramural Research and Division of Research Grants)

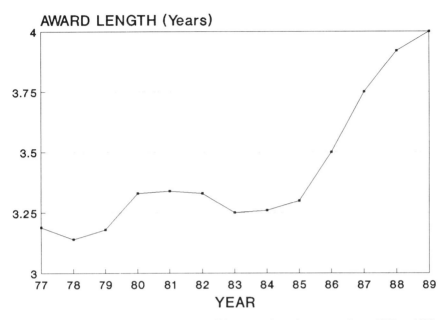

FIGURE 4-20   Average award length for R01 research project grants from 1977 to 1989. (Appendix Table A-15)

has responded to this concern by establishing the FIRST program, which provides 5 years of support for young investigators. For midcareer investigators NIH's Method to Extend Research in Time (MERIT) award can extend the period of grant support up to 10 years. NIH and ADAMHA study sections and advisory councils also have been encouraged to fund proposals for the requested length of the project rather than cutting grant periods. In doing so, future budget obligations of NIH and ADAMHA increased. However, providing stability for investigators over extended periods of time must be weighed against a more flexible system with shorter periods of support.

Multiple Awards

The committee discussed at length principal investigators having multiple grant awards. An analysis of principal investigators receiving R01 grant awards revealed a slight trend toward multiple awards. Between 1978 and 1989 the total number of R01 research project grants grew from 11,929 to 16,084 (Table 4-2). However, of the 4,000 net increase in awards, about 25 percent were awarded to principal investigators already receiving R01 grant support. Thus, the number of principal investigators grew only by

3,000—from 10,200 to 13,200. In this same period, the average number of awards per awardee grew as well—from 1.168 to 1.218.

The reasons for multiple awards are complex. However, the committee feels that, in many instances, investigators may need more than one grant for their research programs. Additionally, the committee believes that intense competition and downward negotiation have forced many investigators to apply for multiple grant awards to avoid funding gaps and to fund their research program fully. The committee also heard speculation that senior investigators with a proven track record of grant support may be listed as the principle investigator to ensure a steady stream of NIH or ADAMHA research grants.

Another confounding aspect of research support is identifying the total number of scientists supported on NIH grants. The NIH data base on grant recipients only includes data on principal investigators. Thus, no data are collected on co-investigators. It is likely that the percent effort on an NIH grant by a co-investigator exceeds that of the principal investigator, who may be dividing his or her time commitments among two or more research grants. Also, junior scientists who may be co-investigators on several projects, but are not principal investigators, may be overlooked by the NIH data base and also by tenure review committees.

There is evidence that the average age of principal investigators is increasing. Between 1979 and 1987 the mean age of investigators supported by ADAMHA increased from 41.5 to 44.6 and from 41.8 to 43.8 for NIH.[19] It is not clear, however, if this has any connection to multiple awards, especially from senior scientists. This may simply reflect the aging of the U.S. population overall. The committee is concerned however, that large blocks of grant funds could be controlled by a few elite scientists, essentially closing the door on young scientists trying to get into the grant system.

R&D CONTRACTS

The NIH enters into contractual agreements to fund R&D in various private and public institutions. Generally, contract proposals are submitted directly to a specific institute in response to Requests for Proposals (RFPs) to develop such research resources as highly specific animal colonies or cell culture lines. The review process for R&D contracts differs from peer review for research grant applications.[3] The requirements of the contract are determined by the institute prior to the announcement of the RFP. Once submitted, the proposals are evaluated by a technical review group within the institute. Finally, senior scientific and contracts management staff evaluate merit and analyze cost considerations.

In 1977 R&D contracts accounted for nearly 20 percent of the extramural budget, but by 1989 allocations for contracts had declined to less than

TABLE 4-2 Recipients of NIH Traditional Research Project (R01) Grants* with Multiple Awards, 1978-1989

| Year | Total Competing and Noncompeting | | | Number of Principal Investigators Having: | | | | | |
| | People | Awards | Awards per Awardee | One Award | | Two Awards | | Three or More Awards | |
				Number	Percent	Number	Percent	Number	Percent
1978	10,211	11,919	1.17	8,723	85.4	1,290	12.6	198	1.9
1979	11,699	13,949	1.19	9,757	83.4	1,677	14.3	265	2.3
1980	12,269	14,691	1.20	10,154	82.8	1,850	15.1	265	2.2
1981	12,342	14,773	1.20	10,227	82.9	1,846	15.0	269	2.2
1982	11,821	14,178	1.20	9,780	82.7	1,781	15.1	260	2.2
1983	12,238	14,844	1.21	9,983	81.6	1,967	16.1	288	2.4
1984	12,452	15,156	1.22	10,137	81.4	1,992	16.0	323	2.6
1985	12,900	15,747	1.22	10,443	81.0	2,118	16.4	339	2.6
1986	13,140	16,015	1.22	10,643	81.0	2,179	16.6	318	2.4
1987	13,277	16,312	1.23	10,653	80.2	2,266	17.1	358	2.7
1988	13,344	16,259	1.22	10,820	81.1	2,185	16.4	339	2.5
1989	13,202	16,084	1.22	10,700	81.0	2,183	16.5	319	2.4

*Does not include supplements.

SOURCE: National Institutes of Health, Division of Research Grants.

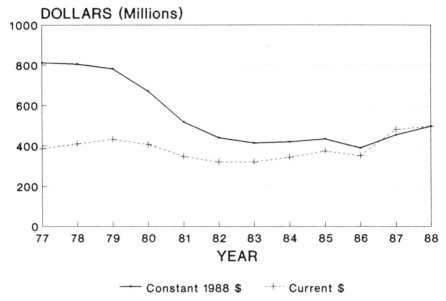

FIGURE 4-21   NIH obligations for research and development contracts from 1977 to 1989. (Appendix Table A-12)

10 percent (Figure 4-9).[11] In constant dollars, NIH obligations to R&D contracts have been halved over this period (Figure 4-21). This shift may have been caused by the stabilization policy's emphasis on grants, where many R&D contracts may have become grants to reach the congressionally mandated quotas.

R&D CENTERS

The NIH supports nearly 600 centers designed to consolidate related research efforts and resources into a single administrative and programmatic structure. Centers serve as well as a vital institutional resource for multidisciplinary research. The funds provided through center grants are used for salaries of key staff, operation of shared resources and services, and center administration. These funds also may be used to recruit new talent to the center, to fund investigators who previously have not obtained competitive peer-reviewed federal funding, to provide interim research support for center investigators, and to obtain new shared resources.

Specialized Centers, Center Core Grants, and General Clinical Research Centers (GCRCs) comprise the bulk of the centers program (Table 4-1). Whereas these centers are primarily for research, other centers support research resources, such as primate and other specialized animal colonies, as well as biotechnology resources. Centers and other research grants, including Biomedical Research and Support Grants, Career Development Awards, and Cooperative Clinical Grants, now account for 18 percent of the NIH extramural budget compared to 22 percent in 1978 (Table 4-1 and Figure 4-9).[11]

The application and review processes for clinical and research centers differ slightly from those of investigator-initiated grant applications. The applicants generally submit a letter of intent. Although the center applications are subjected to peer review by the appropriate institute, the review process also commonly involves site visits. Criteria for review include interdisciplinary coordination, commitment of parent institution, qualifications of the director, impact of the center on the knowledge in the field, staff expertise and needs, shared resources needs, and the quality of the research protocols that will be performed in the center.[20]

The GCRC program is designed to support defined areas within academic medical centers dedicated to patient-related research. These centers can be composed of specialized in-patient and out-patient facilities, laboratories and equipment, and mainframe computers. These are staffed by specialized personnel, such as biostatisticians, computer systems managers, research nurses and dieticians, and research laboratory technicians.

The GCRCs have been instrumental in collecting and analyzing data in vaccine-related clinical research for several bacterial and viral immunogens, and they have provided the infrastructure for the major efforts underway to perform clinical investigations on AIDS. In fact, budget increases since 1986 for the GCRC program were earmarked almost entirely for AIDS research (Judith Vaitukaitus, personal communication). However, the number of GCRCs supported dropped from 93 in 1970 to 78 in 1988, and budget allocations to the GCRCs over this period do not reflect any real growth (Figure 4-22).

In 1989 the IOM undertook a study on NCI's Center Core Grant program.[20] These core grants provide about 20 percent of NCI's grant support in cancer center institutions. By maintaining cohorts of specialized research scientists and clinicians, the centers are successful in obtaining funds from other federal agencies and nonprofit organizations. Whereas the number of centers supported by NCI has stabilized since the late 1970s, budget allocations have declined continuously when measured in constant 1988 dollars (Figure 4-23). The IOM cancer study committee concluded that the NCI centers program would be in serious jeopardy if measures were not taken to reverse the continual erosion of funding for centers. This study committee recommended the following:

- The NCI should strengthen its core support of cancer centers in order to exploit fully the application of these advances in the prevention and treatment of cancer and its consequences.

• The director of NCI should take immediate steps to avert a crisis in the funding of the program during the 1989 fiscal year. The committee recommended further that the directors of NCI and NIH, with the secretary of DHHS, work with the appropriate committees of Congress to develop an adequate budget for the program's 1990 fiscal year.

• The NCI should develop a systematic program plan to ensure adequate fiscal, managerial, and organizational resources; coordination with related programs; and effective scientific oversight for the cancer centers program.

• The director of the NCI should consider how best to increase representation of the cancer centers program in NCI planning and decision-making processes, including regular representation of the centers at the NCI executive committee meetings and creation of an external advisory committee to review their multidisciplinary programs.

• The director of the NCI should strengthen substantially the management capabilities of the cancer centers program unit. That unit must be able to plan, monitor, evaluate, and implement the cancer centers program adequately.

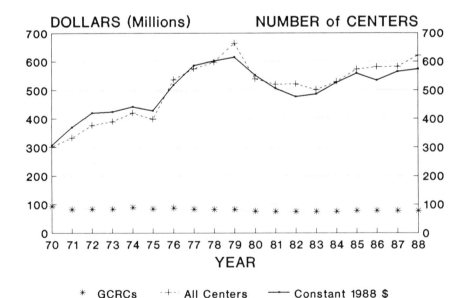

FIGURE 4-22 NIH support for research centers from 1970 to 1988. (Appendix Table A-16)

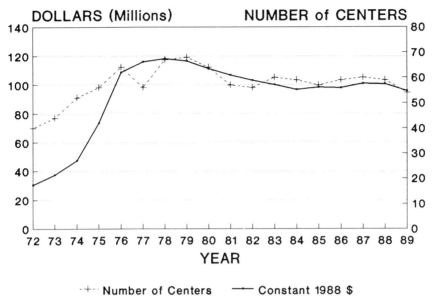

-+- Number of Centers   —•— Constant 1988 $

FIGURE 4-23   National Cancer Institute support for cancer centers from 1972 to 1989. (Appendix Table A-17)

RESEARCH ADMINISTRATION

Grants Management—The Florida Demonstration Project

As the federally sponsored research system has grown and aged, it has acquired a myriad of administrative, managerial, and financial procedures. These procedures seemed necessary and appropriate at the time the sponsored programs began or when they were recommended by Congress, federal agencies, state governments, universities, and participating scientists and engineers. Although all of these groups contributed to the accretion of bureaucratic requirements, there has been a recent movement by them to try to increase efficiency and productivity in all sectors of the American economy, including the research sector.

A model program, designated Phase I of the Florida Demonstration Project (FDP), therefore was designed to test the efficacy of standardizing and simplifying the financial and administrative requirements of grants as a means of enhancing research productivity.[21,22] This program was intended to reduce the administrative burden on grantees by streamlining procedures and reducing costs in the sponsored project system. The demonstration began in April 1986 and ended in December 1987. Nine campuses of the Florida State University System and Miami University participated in the demonstration along with five federal agencies: the Department of

Agriculture, the Department of Energy, NIH, the Office of Naval Research, and the National Science Foundation.

At the outset there were four primary program objectives: (1) standardize postaward administration of federal research grants among the federal agencies to the extent possible; (2) eliminate most federal prior approvals for budget reallocation; (3) simplify research project management procedures; and (4) allow an investigator's collective research program to be one administrative and accounting unit rather than separate units. However, many elements of the sponsored project system were to remain intact, such as the basic framework for federal stewardship and accountability, and there were to be no changes in the federal agencies' project proposal, proposal review and evaluation, and project award mechanisms, and methods for reimbursement of direct and indirect costs.

The Government-University-Industry Research Roundtable (GUIRR) of the National Academy of Sciences was primarily responsible for developing the FDP. The FDP was evaluated initially in August 1986, followed by two questionnaire evaluations in November 1986 and April 1987.[22] These evaluations of the project showed the following results: (1) less time was needed for final action on such project management items as extensions, budget changes, and travel changes; (2) paperwork and administrative tasks decreased throughout the system; (3) principal investigators had more flexibility, responsibility, and control, which the investigators believed increased their own laboratory productivity; (4) federal sponsoring agencies showed a greater trust in the universities' administrative capabilities; (5) relationships between the principal investigators and university administrators as well as between university and federal administrators improved; and (6) scientific and financial accountability were maintained.

The project now has entered Phase II and has been redesignated the Federal Demonstration Project. Twenty-six institutions have been added to the original ten for further evaluation of this project, which began October 1, 1988.

Biomedical Research Support Grants

One program that is tied closely to NIH research project grant awards is the Biomedical Research Support Grant (BRSG) program sponsored by the National Center for Research Resources (formerly known as the Division of Research Resources). Unlike the investigator-initiated research projects that are awarded through a competitive system using peer review, BRSGs are awarded to institutions according to a formula. Rather than requiring institutions to submit proposals for specific projects, the BRSG program provides funds to those research institutions engaged heavily in biomedical research. Thus, the BRSG program provides proportionately more funds (up to a maximum of $500,000) to institutions that previously have demonstrated the strength of their research efforts through the competitive grants system. The flexibility accorded the institution in determining the use of the funds is the unique characteristic of the BRSG program. Recipient institutions are required to have a designated program director, to have an advisory committee to oversee use of the funds, and to advertise the availability of these funds within the institution. With the exception of a few minor restrictions, the use of the funds is left to the discretion of the institution. Many institutions establish peer review panels to evaluate proposals requesting BRSG funds for research or shared equipment. The latitude granted to the institutions for the use of these funds gives them more flexibility to fund emerging areas of research or new investigators before they can be fully competitive in the traditional research project grant (R01) system.

The BRSG program has come under increasing attack in the budget preparation process over the past few years and has been identified as one program to trim in order to reduce the NIH budget. In fact, the program was trimmed from $55 million in 1989 to $44 million in 1990. It is slated for yet deeper cuts in the 1991 budget, in which only $17 million is allocated to the program. It is not clear to the committee why there have been repeated attempts to eliminate this program. The committee can only speculate that NIH may not favor local control of these funds, which are not subject to national peer review. However, the committee strongly endorses this program because it allows all institutions to enhance their own health research programs according to institutional needs. The BRSG program may be an increasingly valuable grant mechanism for maintaining career stability for mid level scientists if the number of research grants awarded becomes more unpredictable.

INCREASING COSTS OF ANIMAL USE

The cost of acquiring and caring for laboratory animals has continued to increase since 1978. In large institutions the costs of maintaining centralized animal facilities usually are included as part of per diem charges for animals. For example, at one university per diem charges for mice rose from 5.5 cents in 1978 to 14 cents in 1987—an increase of over 150 percent—while the Consumer Price Index rose by 74.1 percent during that time. Over the same period, the per diem charges increased for dogs (from $3.60 to $8.61), for monkeys ($1.05 to $2.71), and for cats (from $1.30 to 3.20).[23] ADAMHA estimated that new regulations concerning animal care would cost in the neighborhood of $40,000 to $70,000 per grant on the care of primates and dogs.[24]

The scientific community is very concerned about the increasingly stringent federal regulations for animal experimentation and the effect these regulations have on the increasing costs of doing research. Pressure from animal rights groups to tighten these regulations has had and will continue to have a profound effect on the numbers and kinds of animals used in health sciences research. Although scientists are actively involved in seeking alternatives to animal testing, they feel certain types of systems biology experimentation must be performed in animals. The committee fears as well that curbing all animal experimentation directly or indirectly by imposing unrealistic regulations will slow scientific progress in fighting human disease.

INDIRECT COST RECOVERY

During World War II, the federal government entered into contractual agreements with research universities in mutually beneficial partnerships. As a result, the government was able to capitalize on research results by supporting scientists at these institutions. Not only were the direct costs of performing the research supported, but the indirect or overhead costs of the research were reimbursed as well. Thus, it became federal policy to reimburse institutions for the ancillary costs of performing federally sponsored research.[25]

The institutional indirect cost rate is negotiated annually on an individual basis with one of the sponsoring federal agencies, and this rate is honored by other agencies sponsoring research at the institution. The Office of Management and Budget circulars A-21 and A-110 set the government-wide accounting principles for direct costs and indirect costs of sponsored research at colleges and universities.[26] The indirect costs are calculated as an average cost of research on a prorated share of all overhead costs in proportion to the ratio of sponsored research expenditures (all sources) to the total expenditures of the university, rather than the marginal costs of a research project. Indirect costs are subdivided into the following seven categories: (1) operation and maintenance expenses, (2) use charges for buildings and equipment, (3) library expenses, (4) sponsored projects administration, (5) general administration, (6) student administration and services, and (7) departmental administration. Whereas the costs associated with the first three categories can be documented, the latter four administrative cost components are the least definitive and most difficult to evaluate in terms of individual research projects. Although the costs associated with operations, maintenance, and use allowance are more easily documented, they are no less controversial in these extremely tight fiscal times.

Before 1966 indirect costs were fixed by Congress. Since then the

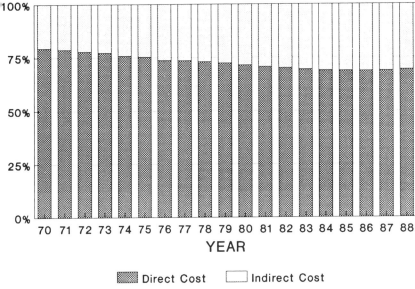

FIGURE 4-24 Proportion of direct and indirect costs for NIH research grants from 1970 to 1988. (Appendix Table A-19)

policy changed, and the average rate has climbed from 25 percent to more than 31 percent for NIH-sponsored research (the range is 7 to 100 percent) (Figure 4-24). This reflects a shift in federal policy from direct support for facilities through facilities grants to a policy of indirect cost recovery. In effect, universities and colleges have been forced to increase indirect cost rates in order to maintain or update facilities. However, individual investigators perceive rising indirect cost rates as a threat to the available pool of funds for the direct costs of health research. Indirect costs for facilities renewal is covered in more detail in Chapter 6.

SUMMARY AND CONCLUSIONS

From this review of the funding trends for the various programs of research support, the committee concluded that the stabilization policy was successful in maintaining support for investigator-initiated research project grants. As a result of the emphasis on research project grants, this portion of the extramural budget grew from 51 to 67 percent between 1977 and 1990, rising from $2.5 billion to $3.9 billion. Consequently, in order to meet increasing annual targets of new and competing grant awards, funds had to be taken from commitments to ongoing research projects as well as by reducing new awards through downward negotiation. Funds also were diverted from other programs—specifically research centers and contracts— and resources for training declined steadily throughout the 1980s.

The committee further concluded that scientists responded to these growing problems by increasing their number of applications to maintain research programs. Although the total number of grants supported has grown from 15,500 to more than 20,000 since 1977, the often-cited award rates and pay lines have dropped steadily over this period. These declines have been caused by several factors including the substantial increase in the volume of applications; and lengthening award periods. These declines also have been caused in part by the fact that study sections have been approving steadily increasing percentages of the applications and assigning increasingly higher (lower-numbered) priority scores.

Additional conclusions were drawn by the committee from an analysis of the effects of the lengthy application and review process for research grants. The review process for new NIH/ADAMHA grant applications takes a minimum of 9 months. Without intermediate feedback steps, those applications requiring modification and resubmission can take as long as 18 months. A misunderstood or poorly written proposal, even if it involves meritorious work, may lead to loss of support for a successful laboratory with important ongoing projects, and although it is technically possible to restore funding by resubmitting amended proposals and clarifying the parts that were unclear, in reality, support has since disappeared. The committee believes that, in these cases, people are fired and the projects halted, and by the time support is later restored, it is often too late to salvage talent and other resources. The committee was concerned that the frailty of this system hinders long-term research planning and can affect career investigators adversely. It also prevents timely work in new areas and in those sectors in which health crises require faster-paced research activities.

Thus, despite the historically unbroken trend of increasing annual funding, the committee concluded that the episodic nature of funding (in terms of interruptions), downward negotiations, and the progressively de-creasing likelihood of receiving awards have fostered perceptions within the academic community that careers in health sciences research are unstable and unpredictable. These perceptions are exacerbated by delays in deter-mining federal budget allocations, fluctuating funding patterns within NIH and ADAMHA, and reductions in awards for ongoing projects. Perhaps partly because of these problems, the length of time that principal inves-tigators receive continuous R01 grant support from the NIH/ADAMHA sponsored research system has been cut in half, from more than 13 years in the 1950s to less than 6 years in the 1980s.

In addition, as the federally sponsored research system has grown and aged, it has acquired a myriad of administrative, managerial, and financial procedures that have increased bureaucratic requirements. The Florida Demonstration Project is commendable in its goal to reduce administrative burdens and increase laboratory productivity of the scientific work force. The committee concluded that health sciences research requires an environment that identifies, encourages, and develops creativity. Such an environment requires stable support for scientists and flexibility in allocating resources to meet changing demands. When the environment is positive, supportive, and reasonably predictable and optimistic, it encourages the recruitment and retention of talented health sciences researchers.

REFERENCES

1. U.S. Department of Health and Human Services; Public Health Service. 1989. NIH Almanac. Publication No. 89-5. Bethesda, Md.: National Institutes of Health.
2. U.S. Department of Health and Human Services; Public Health Service. 1989. NIH Data Book Publication No. 90-1261. Bethesda, Md.: National Institutes of Health.
3. U.S. Department of Health and Human Services; Public Health Service. 1988. ADAMHA Funding Mechanisms for Grants and Awards. Rockville, Md.: Alcohol, Drug Abuse, and Mental Health Administration.
4. Seggel, R.L. 1985. Stabilizing the Funding of NIH and ADAMHA Research Project Grants. Washington, D.C.: National Academy Press.
5. U.S. Department of Health and Human Services; Public Health Service. ADAMHA Data Source Book, FY 1988. ADAMHA Program Analysis Report No. 89-18. Rockville, Md.: Alcohol, Drug Abuse, and Mental Health Administration.
6. Institute of Medicine. 1988. A Healthy NIH Intramural Program: Structural Change or Administrative Remedies? Washington, D.C.: National Academy Press.
7. U.S. Department of Health, Education, and Welfare; Public Health Service. 1976. Report of the President's Biomedical Research Panel. DHEW Publication No. (OS)76-500. Washington, D.C.
8. Institute of Medicine. 1979. DHEW's Research Planning Principles: A Review. Washington, D.C.: National Academy of Sciences.
9. Institute of Medicine. 1980. DHEW Health Research Planning, Phase II: A Review. Washington, D.C.: National Academy of Sciences.
10. Moskowitz, Jay; Associate Director for Science Policy and Legislation, National Institutes of Health. 1989. Presentation at AAAS Symposia on Research and Development in the FY 1990 Federal Budget. Washington, D.C.: April 1989.
11. U.S. Department of Health and Human Services. 1988. Extramural Trends, FY 1978-87. Bethesda, Md.: National Institutes of Health, Division of Research Grants.
12. U.S. Department of Health and Human Services; Public Health Service. 1985. DRG Peer Review Trends; Workload and Actions of DRG Study Sections, 1975-1985. Bethesda, Md.: National Institutes of Health.
13. U.S. Department of Health and Human Services; Public Health Service. 1986. DRG Peer Review Trends; Member Characterisitcs: DRG Study Sections, Institute Review Groups, Advisory Councils and Boards, 1977-1986. Bethesda, Md.: National Institutes of Health.
14. U.S. Department of Health and Human Services; Public Health Service. 1988. The health of biomedical research institutions: Report of the regional meetings. Proceedings of the 57th Meeting of the Advisory Committee to the Director, National Institutes of Health, Bethesda, Md. June 27-28, 1988.

15. U.S. Department of Health and Human Services; Public Health Service. 1988. NIH Advisory Committees: Authority, Structure, Function, Members. Publication No. 88-11. Bethesda, Md.: National Institutes of Health.
16. U.S. General Accounting Office: Biomedical Research: Issues Related to Increasing Size of NIH Grant Awards. Report No. GAO/HRD-88-90BR; May 1988.
17. U.S. Department of Health and Human Services; Public Health Service. 1985. Academic Research Equipment and Equipment Needs in the Biological and Medical Sciences. NIH Program Evaluation Report No. 85-2769. Bethesda, Md.: National Institutes of Health.
18. U.S. Department of Health and Human Services; Public Health Service. 1984. The extramural awards system. Proceedings of the 50th Meeting of the Advisory Committee to the Director, National Institutes of Health, Bethesda, Md. November 19, 1984.
19. U.S. Department of Health and Human Services, Public Health Service: Age Trends of ADAMHA Principal Investigators. ADAMHA Program Analysis Report, No. 88-10. Rockville, Md.: Alcohol, Drug Abuse, and Mental Health Administration.
20. Institute of Medicine. 1989. A Stronger Cancer Centers Program. Washington, D.C.: National Academy Press.
21. Hively, W. 1988. Getting rid of red tape. American Scientist 76:241-244.
22. National Academy of Sciences; Government-University-Research Roundtable. 1988. Unpublished evaluation documents.
23. National Research Council. 1988. Use of Laboratory Animals in Biomedical and Behavioral Research. Washington, D.C.: National Academy Press.
24. Holden, C. 1989. A preemptive strike for animal research. Science 244:415-416.
25. Association of American Universities. 1988. Indirect Costs Associated with Federal Support on University Campuses: Some Suggestions for Change (Draft). Washington, D.C.: AAU Ad Hoc Committee on the Indirect Costs to the Executive Committee of the AAU.
26. Office of Management and Budget: Principles for Determining Costs Applicable to Grants, Contracts, and Other Agreements with Educational Institutions. OMB Circular A-21. Washington, D.C. (Revised February 1979.)

5

Nurturing Scientific Talent

Maintaining a cadre of highly talented health scientists is the most critical element in sustaining the vitality of the U.S. system of health sciences research. Evidence from across the educational spectrum indicates that the United States is facing a future shortage of qualified researchers, which will threaten the nation's ability to prepare for scientific challenges of the twenty-first century. In the next 15 years many of the individuals who conceived the ideas that have revolutionized health sciences research will be retiring. Neglect in educating and training their replacements inevitably will lead to a decline in the nation's capabilities in health-related research, an area in which the United States has maintained an unchallenged world leadership for the past 40 years.

Particularly alarming is the apparent decline in the number of physicians engaged in health-related research. The study of many fundamental biological questions begins with investigation into human disease processes, and human data are essential to address these questions effectively. The defining and understanding of these problems are largely in the hands of physician-scientists, who also serve as technology-transfer agents, translating fundamental laboratory discoveries into clinical practice.

Accurately assessing the magnitude and timing of an impending personnel shortage depends upon a variety of factors. Scientific employment growth in academia, government, and the private sector is tied closely to the economic health of the nation. As the post-World War II baby boomers grow older, the retirement rate among scientists trained in the 1950s and 1960s will accelerate, increasing the demand for replacements. Also, a higher death rate in this more elderly scientist population will increase demand in the health scientist labor market. The composition of the future health scientist work force also will be affected by changing demographics with regard to age, gender, race, ethnicity, and immigration, as well as the quality of scientific education and training.

An accurate assessment of all of these factors affecting the scientific work force must be part of a decision-making process regarding research training needs. A comprehensive talent renewal plan must encompass the multitude of research disciplines that range from basic to applied investigation. This chapter examines the available data on the research work force and highlights the possible implications for the future health scientist talent pool.

PROBLEMS IN THE HUMAN RESOURCE BASE

Precollege

The pathway to a scientific career does not begin in undergraduate or postgraduate years; rather, an interest in science is kindled in the early years of formal education—kindergarten through grade 12. However, several recent national and international studies have shown a continuous decline in science and mathematics skills by American students at all educational levels. Although the committee focused its deliberations on the resources for graduate and postdoctoral education and training, the committee recognized that competency in precollege and undergraduate science and mathematics education is critical for preparing students for scientific careers. Additionally, an early appreciation of the excitement of scientific discovery is important for attracting students into scientific careers.

About three-quarters of all students who eventually major in science and engineering follow a college preparatory curriculum.[1] However, the National Assessment of Educational Progress, which is part of the federally sponsored Nation's Report Card conducted by the Educational Testing Service, concluded that only 7 percent of 17 year olds in 1986 were prepared adequately for college-level science courses.[2] This report also confirmed the race and ethnicity gaps that previous studies have found in science achievement. Whereas only about 15 percent of African-American and Hispanic 17 year olds demonstrated the ability to analyze scientific procedures and data, nearly half of their white peers could do so.

Despite inherent difficulties in interpreting comparative international education data, a study of mathematics and science abilities among students in four foreign countries, four Canadian provinces, and the United States ranked the American students near the bottom in these skills.[3] The National

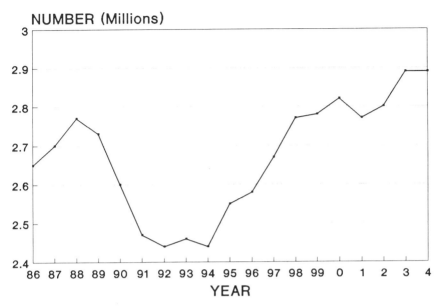

NUMBER (Millions)

YEAR

FIGURE 5-1 Projected number of U.S. high school graduates from 1986 to 2004. (Reprinted with permission from Western Interstate Commission for Higher Education. High School Graduates: Projections by State, 1986 to 2004. Boulder, CO; 1988.)

Research Council has drawn attention to the poor mathematics proficiency of American students in a report entitled *Everybody Counts: A Report to the Nation on the Future of Mathematics Education.*[4] This study called for a complete overhaul of precollege mathematics education in the United States and suggested alternative educational strategies to counteract this growing problem.

Moreover, national demographic evidence indicates that the number of high school graduates is expected to decline by 12 percent between 1988 and 1992, from nearly 2.77 million to 2.44 million students (Figure 5-1).[5] Unless these trends change, the declining number of high school graduates is expected to lead to declining undergraduate enrollment in U.S. colleges and universities in the early to mid 1990s. However, the number of high school graduates is expected to return to the 1988 level by 1998 and will coincide directly with a rapidly increasing retirement rate of university faculty.

Undergraduate

A recent study by the Office of Technology Assessment, tracking the progress of American students toward careers in science and engineering, exemplifies the attrition rates from the available talent pool during all stages of scientific career development.[6] From an original study group of 4,000 ninth-grade students, only 1,000 had sufficient mathematics abilities at that point to pursue a scientific or engineering career. When these students had completed their secondary school education, only 500 were adequately prepared to continue in a science or engineering college curriculum. At this point, women were represented equally in the study group. However, upon entering college the number of women electing to pursue a science or engineering career fell to 44 of 250 individuals compared to 140 of 250 for men. By the completion of their baccalaureate programs, only 66 of the original study group of 4,000 received B.S. degrees—a precipitous drop of more than 98 percent in the original. This example illustrates vividly the problem of recruiting individuals into the sciences, especially as it applies to women and other underrepresented groups.

Unfortunately, major losses in the science and engineering talent pool occur during the undergraduate years.[7] Students usually make career decisions during this critical undergraduate period. Thus, recruiting individuals into the health sciences will depend upon the following factors:

- enthusiasm engendered by high-quality teaching,
- scientific opportunity and excitement,
- economic status of the nation,
- financial support for education, and
- financial rewards from employment opportunities.

Students interested in health sciences research generally follow curricula that prepare them for graduate study leading to professional degrees—either Ph.D.s or M.D.s. Relevant areas include not only biology and chemistry but also such fields as physics, mathematics, psychology, or the social sciences. Data gathered over the past 10 years reveal a decline in earned bachelor degrees in the life sciences (Figure 5-2).[7,8] Although life scientists are not the exclusive talent pool for the health sciences, the committee believes that a significant portion of health scientists with advanced degrees come from this student population. Also, the committee believes that over the last 10 to 15 years, the supply of high-quality graduate students in the health sciences has declined.

Considerable discussion has focused on reasons for the failure of science educators to stimulate student interest in scientific careers. The committee believes that this failure may be due partly to the widespread practice of collegiate science education stressing passive learning through lectures rather than active learning through participation in research. Honors programs that include hands-on research in conjunction with faculty mentors provide an example of active learning that can stimulate students

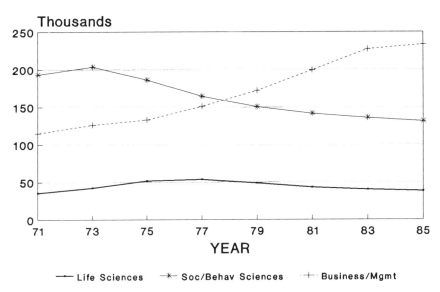

FIGURE 5-2 Number of bachelors degrees awarded in the life sciences, social and behavioral sciences, and business/management from 1965 to 1985.[3]

to pursue research careers. Also, family values concerning education have a great deal of influence on childhood learning and performance.

Although science education and training for undergraduates fall within the purview of the Science and Engineering Education Directorate of the National Science Foundation (NSF), the problem of recruiting students into science and engineering careers has recently been addressed by Congress. The National Science Scholars Program, part of the President's Educational Excellence Act, is designed to encourage exceptional students to pursue careers in scientific and engineering fields.[9] Modeled on congressional appointments to military academies, the proposed program calls for federal support for undergraduate education in science and engineering for two appointees (one female and one male) for every member of Congress. The awards would be 4-year fellowships, based on merit and a competitive selection process, for study at an institution of the student's choice. The program would sponsor approximately 1,000 new scholarships per year, each having an annual stipend of $5,000. Totaling $18 million per year when fully operational, this program should act as a catalyst to attract additional student financial aid from other sources. The committee believes that this type of program focuses local attention on science and engineering education and serves as a highly visible example of congressional support for renewing scientific talent. The small size of this program, however, clearly will not be sufficient to meet expected shortages in all of the sciences. The racial and ethnic composition of the U.S. population is changing, and these changes also will affect the pool from which scientific talent is drawn. The U.S. Bureau of the Census estimates that the minority composition of the 22-year-old population will grow to 20 percent by 2005— up from 14 percent in 1975.[10] Ethnic and racial minorities historically have been underrepresented in science and engineering. Whereas nearly 5 percent of white and Asian 22 year olds have earned baccalaureate degrees in natural science or engineering, only 1.6 percent of blacks, Hispanics, and Native Americans have earned the same degrees.[11]

In the 1970s the National Institutes of Health (NIH) created the Minority Access to Research Careers (MARC) Honors Program to increase the number of minority students pursuing graduate study leading to a Ph.D. in biomedical science. The largest portion of the MARC program is the Honors Undergraduate Research Training Program. Trainees at selected institutions receive tuition support and a stipend to participate in a specially structured curriculum. Working closely with faculty members on laboratory research projects in the biomedical sciences is a key element in the training experience. Longitudinal data are not yet substantial enough to determine if this program is having a significant effect on recruiting minorities into graduate health research programs, however. Although the Institute of Medicine (IOM) undertook a survey evaluation of the MARC program in 1985, it was too early to gauge the success of the program, and no remedies were suggested to address the problems identified.[12]

Scientific Doctorates (Ph.D.s)

The transition from undergraduate to graduate school is another critical juncture in the retention of candidates for future careers in the health sciences. Large numbers of undergraduates elect not to pursue graduate studies; of those who do, an unknown number either may not complete their graduate program or may leave research upon earning a doctorate. Data from the NSF Survey of Graduate Science and Engineering Students and Postdoctorates reveal that graduate student enrollment (not including postdoctorates) in the life sciences has grown only slightly since 1980, from 102,504 to 108,641, whereas enrollment in the physical sciences has grown by more than 23 percent annually, from 26,952 to 33,203.[13] Enrollment in the social sciences has declined slightly over the same period, from 94,778 to 91,884.[13]

There is a considerable lag time affecting the scientific labor market that must be considered when policy is formulated. Presently recognized opportunities will affect the scientific work force 5 to 8 years hence, upon completion of a doctoral program, clinical training program, or a postdoctoral fellowship. In short, salaries and economic opportunity in 1989 will have affected graduate enrollment that year, but the 1989 graduate school entrants will not affect labor force supply until possibly 1995. This scenario is compounded by the fact that there also will be a significant decline in the size of the 18- to 24-year-old population—the talent pool available for recruiting into graduate study—in the late 1990s, when many tenured faculty members are expected to retire.[8]

The number of foreign graduate students enrolled in U.S. institutions as well as the percent of degrees conferred on foreign nationals has increased steadily over the past decade.[14,15] The United States produces nearly 14,500 natural scientists and engineers annually, up from 12,000 in 1978. In 1987 about 9,700 science and engineering doctorates were conferred on U.S. citizens or foreign nationals with permanent visas. The remaining 3,800 doctorates were conferred on foreign citizens with temporary U.S. visas. Of those students on temporary visas receiving doctorates in 1987, about half remained in the United States to pursue employment (23 percent) or postdoctoral studies (25 percent). Thus, immigration compensates for shortages in trained U.S. personnel and adds to the intellectual and technological abilities of the country's scientific work force. But while foreign students earned only 16 percent of the doctorates in life sciences in 1987, the committee believes that the health sciences should not follow the path of engineering, in which almost half of the doctorates are conferred on foreign nationals. Such heavy reliance on foreign talent could jeopardize the future success of American science efforts and the national economy should fewer and fewer degree recipients elect to remain in the United States.

Although women make up 42 percent of the U.S. work force (U.S. Department of Labor Statistics, personal communication, 10-19-89) they have been underrepresented historically in science and engineering.[16] In 1977 women represented only 10.4 percent of all doctoral scientists and engineers.[17] Although their numbers have grown—from 31,800 in 1977 to 73,423 in 1987, for example—women scientists and engineers still account for only 16.3 percent of the total doctoral population. However, the annual proportion of doctorates conferred on women has been growing steadily over the last three decades.[15] In 1987 women earned 35 percent of the doctorates awarded in the life sciences. In the social sciences they earned 43 percent, but they earned only 17 percent of all doctorates in the physical sciences. Since individuals in each of these broad categories pursue careers in the health sciences, these data indicate that there have been small gains toward equal representation between men and women in the scientific work force.

The proportion of non-Asian minorities receiving doctorates is not increasing; rather, recruitment appears to be worsening in these groups.[15] Whereas the number of black women earning doctorates annually between 1977 and 1987 has remained fairly steady at about 500, the number of degrees conferred annually on black men has been halved—to about 300. Also, whereas doctorates conferred on Hispanic women have more than doubled—to 286—in the same period, the number going to Hispanic men has remained steady at about 300. These data raise serious questions about policies and programs for improving minority participation in higher education as well as research and pose a problem regarding cultural values. The committee emphasizes that the recruiting difficulties of non-Asian minority males should be of particular concern to all policymakers and educators.

The United States employs about 12,500 new Ph.D. scientists and engineers each year.[18] Industry has been creating about 5,500 new Ph.D. positions per year for scientists and engineers. If these hiring practices prevail and retirements in this sector begin to increase as we approach the year 2000, the demand in industry and business could increase to nearly 9,500 by that time. Retirement rates of academic faculty also are expected to increase over the next 15 years, rising from about 2,000 in 1988 to more than 4,500 in 2004. Although demographic evidence indicates that there may be a dearth in undergraduate enrollment in the early 1990s, the impending retirements, coinciding with a surge of 18 to 24 year olds toward the end of the next decade could create an annual academic demand for new Ph.D. scientists and engineers of nearly 8,500 by 2004. At current production rates, even if we rely heavily on the possibility of filling positions with foreign students receiving U.S. doctorates, the annual shortfall still may be as high as 7,500 in the first decade of the twenty-first century.[18] Although these data predict shortages for all natural sciences and for engineering, potential shortages in the health sciences can be expected as well.

Data from the Doctorate Records Survey shows that between 1973 and 1987, employment of biomedical scientists by all sectors grew 4.9 percent annually, rising from 43,000 to 84,500. This includes the 43,000 scientists and 8,200 postdoctorates employed by academic institutions regardless of their level of research activity, 16,000 scientists employed by industry, as well as other Ph.D.s outside academia actively engaged in or managing research and development.

Seventy-six percent of these scientists hold doctorates in biomedical sciences (Figure 5-3); the remaining twenty-four percent have doctorates in fields other than biomedical science. Over this same period the annual output of new biomedical Ph.D. recipients grew by 12.8 percent—from 3,520 to 3,969. However, not all recipients of biomedical degrees are employed as biomedical scientists; approximately 24 percent are engaged in other activities (Figure 5-4). Over the past decade the growth in employment for

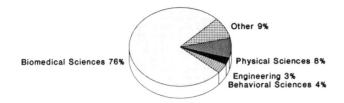

Degree Types as a Percent
of the Workforce

FIGURE 5-3 Composition of the biomedical work force. (Source: Office of Science and Engineering Personnel, National Research Council)

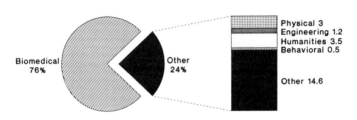

Field of Employment

FIGURE 5-4 Employment of biomedical scientists. (Source: Office of Science and Engineering Personnel, National Research Council)

biomedical scientists largely has been in industry, growing an average of 12 to 13 percent annually.[19]

The employment of behavioral scientists grew 113.6 percent between 1973 and 1987, rising from 31,669 to 67,651.[19] More than 91 percent of the vacancies in behavioral sciences are filled by individuals with doctorates in the behavioral sciences. The number of behavioral sciences doctoral degrees conferred annually has climbed from 3,542 to 3,960, reflecting an 11.8 percent change over the same period. One element that may skew these data is the surge in clinical psychology degrees that has occurred over the past few years.

One factor affecting the output of Ph.D. scientists is the increasing time needed to earn a doctorate.[20] Whereas the median registered time to degree (i.e., the time the student is registered for formal courses or thesis preparation with the university registrar) for all fields was about 5.4 years in 1967, by 1987 it had increased to 6.9 years. While the largest increase was noted for graduate students in the humanities, doctoral candidates in the physical and life sciences now spend more than 6 years in graduate study, compared to just over 5 years two decades ago. In the social sciences the median was 7.2 years in the 1987 survey, compared to 5.2 years in

1967. It is not clear to the committee how this affects the financial support mechanisms from the federal government or other sources.

Professional Doctorates (M.D.s and M.D./Ph.D.s)

Physician-scientists are charged with carrying fundamental discoveries in the laboratory to the patient and assessing the efficacy of new treatments and other interventions for improved health care. The recruitment of physician-scientists into research careers is hampered severely by the length of time necessary for clinical training, the often unfocused structure of clinical research experience, the need for the individual to understand increasingly complex technologies, and the requirement of the physician to generate clinical income at the expense of time for performing research. At a time when biology and medicine offer exciting opportunities for improved health care, this declining interest in investigative careers is particularly troublesome. The problem is magnified for the fields of public health and preventive medicine, where no practice income is raised to support salaries or subsidize education.

The majority of M.D. and M.D./Ph.D. scientists are employed by medical schools, the government, and private research institutions. According to the American Medical Association (AMA) Physician Masterfile, there were 569,160 federal and nonfederal physicians in the United States as of December 1986.[21] Of these, 86,670 (15.2 percent) were female and 123,090 (21.6 percent) were foreign medical graduates (excluding Canadian graduates). The number of physicians reporting research activity had grown from 11,929 in 1970 to 18,535 in 1983. However, from the time of the 1983 survey to 1986, there was a drop of nearly 700—to 17,847 physicians engaged in research.[21] This also reflects a drop from 3.6 percent of the total physician population engaged in research in 1983 to 3.1 percent in 1986. The 1986 population of physician researchers was composed of 16.2 percent women and 23.5 percent foreign medical graduates, both groups being represented slightly higher than their proportion in the total physician population. Although these data may be flawed and the small shifts reported by the AMA may not be significant, the committee believes that in recent years there has been no growth in the number of physicians participating in research.

The number of applicants to U.S. medical schools has dropped by more than 30 percent in the past 10 years, from 40,600 in 1977 to 28,100 in 1987 (Figure 5-5).[22,23] This decline has engendered concern in the nation's medical centers about the future quality of medical care in the United States as well as the capabilities of physician-scientists.

With the increasing sophistication of health sciences research, educators have recognized the need to develop pathways to ensure that physicians

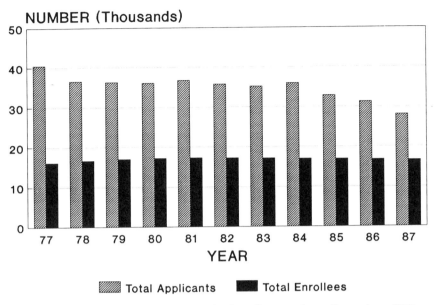

FIGURE 5-5   Number of U.S. medical school applicants and enrollment from 1977 to 1988.[22,23]

are as rigorously trained in scientific methodology as their Ph.D. counterparts. One pathway for achieving this goal is to encourage some physicians to enter doctoral programs in specific research areas leading to a combined M.D./Ph.D. degree. While more than 100 of the 127 U.S. medical schools offer programs for combined M.D./Ph.D. degrees in various areas such as biomedical sciences, social sciences, humanities, biomedical engineering, and law, and only 20 to 30 graduate significant numbers of M.D./Ph.D. candidates.[23] Such combined training provides enhanced research experience that more thoroughly prepares physician researchers for independent basic or clinical investigation.

Some committee members believe that although M.D./Ph.D. programs provide a suitable model for training physicians in research methodology, these are not the pathways followed by most physicians pursuing careers as independent investigators. There are existing models in the nonbiological sciences that tailor coursework in areas to meet the special needs of the physician-scientist, and that link supervision with an established physician mentor (e.g., the Robert Wood Johnson Clinical Scholars Program). For physicians who choose investigative careers in disciplines such as epidemiology, health services research, or health policy, these alternative models may be preferred.

From Degree to Scientist

The prolonged period of time it takes to earn a doctorate and the subsequent extensive postdoctorate training time necessary for both Ph.D. and M.D. scientists often force these individuals to postpone at least some aspects of their personal lives. Both the financial concerns of young families and the balancing needs of two-career families encourage these scientists to move more quickly to establish a stable career.

Clinical training is of particular concern because it requires a substantial time investment, especially if the physician embarks on a career requiring subspecialization. Subspecialties in internal medicine and surgery now require between 5 to 7 years of postdoctoral training after medical school. Since many specialty boards do not allow credit toward certification for research, a formal research training period most often following the clinical subspecialty training, extends the training time invested to 8 or more years. This training time often coincides with the payback period of the considerable financial debt that many physician graduates accumulate during medical school.

Moreover, because of clinical training demands, research training experiences for physician-scientists often are unstructured and poorly focused. It is rare for either clinical training or clinical research experiences to include formal instruction in scientific design, research methodology, and statistical analysis. Additionally, if they lack critical review or accreditation, clinical research training programs fail to introduce standards and accountability. As a result, physician-scientists often are less prepared for pursuing research than more rigorously trained Ph.D. scientists who have had 4 to 5 years of formal research laboratory training. A 2-year research experience, particularly when poorly focused, often leaves physician-scientists less prepared for competing in the peer-reviewed grant system than are more formally trained Ph.D. scientists.

Other pressures in the modern medicine environment add to the discouragement of physicians involved in clinical investigation as well. A recent IOM report on resources for clinical investigation concluded that fundamental changes in the organization of health care and the mounting efforts aimed at cost containment discourage clinical research scientists from pursuing clinical investigations.[24] Along with the pressures that young physician-scientists face early in their careers, there are pressures upon all physicians to earn clinical income for their academic health center. Clinical income is more predictable than research grants, particularly in terms of institutional revenues. As medical schools rely more and more on faculty practice plans for salary support, clinical faculty members are pressured to maintain their clinical practice incomes. These pressures—direct or indirect, bold or subtle—are felt by virtually all M.D. investigators.

Compounding these difficulties, the practice of medicine has become more complex and uses more advanced technology than ever before. Even the so-called cognitive specialties such as internal medicine are heavily dependent upon advanced technological procedures, which require technical skills that must be practiced regularly to maintain a high level of competence, making it more difficult for physician-scientists to devote precious time to scientific investigation (unless these individuals are in unusually supportive academic environments).

PROBLEMS WITH THE FINANCIAL SUPPORT BASE

For nearly 40 years the Science and Engineering Education (SEE) Directorate of NSF has been the primary sponsor of programs for developing scientific talent at the undergraduate level. At its peak in 1960 and 1961, this directorate controlled more than 40 percent of the NSF budget.[25] In the ensuing 20 years, appropriations to SEE failed to keep pace with other parts of the NSF budget, until only 1.5 percent was allocated to science and engineering education by 1983. In recent years, however, the administration has recognized the vital importance of science and engineering to national security and international competitiveness. This reemphasis is reflected in the recent NSF budgets where funding to SEE has grown from $55 million in 1987 to a proposed $251 million in 1991—nearly 10 percent of the 1991 NSF budget.

Federal support for training health scientists began with the passage of the National Cancer Act of 1937 which authorized the U.S. Surgeon General to provide fellowships and train personnel for cancer research and prevention. This authority was expanded in the Public Health Service Act of 1944, expanding training programs sponsored by the NIH. This act not only increased the research capacity of the U.S., but also provided broad financial support to medical students, whether or not they expected to pursue research careers. In 1973 the Nixon administration impounded NIH training funds in an effort to phase out all research training. Congress responded by passing the National Research Service Award (NRSA) Act (P.L. 93-348) in 1974. This act authorized training at the level of the Public Health Service to be conducted primarily in the NIH, the Alcohol, Drug Abuse, and Mental Health Administration (ADAMHA), and the Health Resources Service Administration (HRSA). By creating a separate authorization, research training is now loosely connected to research but the budgets are acted upon separately by congressional appropriations committees.

The NRSA act eliminated support for medical students except those pursuing research careers. Additionally, the act included a service obligation requiring those trainees receiving funds to be actively engaged in

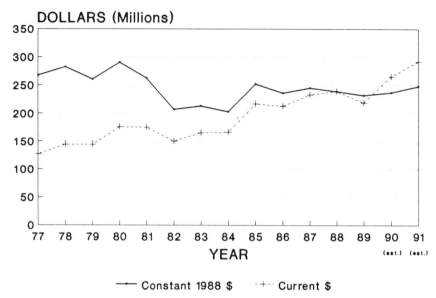

FIGURE 5-6 NIH obligations for National Research Service Award (NRSA) training.
(Appendix Table A-12)

research equivalent to one month of service for each month of support.
This requirement has been modified to allow for short periods of support
without a payback. However, if trainees elect not to pursue research careers they must pay back the costs of their education to the government.
The NRSA act limited support to an aggregate of 5 years for predoctoral
studies and 3 years for postdoctoral research.

The NIH and ADAMHA are the primary federal sponsors for training
in the health sciences. In 1971 NIH allocations for training as a percent
of R&D funds exceeded 18 percent.[26] Research training allocations fell
below 11 percent of the NIH research budget in 1973 and have continued
to decline, accounting for less than 5 percent of R&D allocations in
1988. Additionally, appropriations targeted for training have declined from
nearly $290 million in 1980 to about $250 million in 1990 when measured
in constant 1988 dollars (Figure 5-6).[27]

The number of full-time training positions (FTTPs) supported by NIH
has remained fairly constant each year—between 11,000 and 12,000—since
the late 1970s (Figure 5-7). However, in order to increase sagging stipend
levels, NIH trimmed support for 1,000 FTTPs in fiscal year 1989.[28] Since
NIH supports approximately one-quarter of the graduate students in the
biomedical sciences through the NRSA program, these cuts in training

positions were quite significant. NIH reestablished these positions by reprogramming other funds in 1989.

Declining training support has devastated the training of the next generation of behavioral and social scientists.[29] In the early 1970s ADAMHA allocations for research training exceeded 14 percent of R&D funds. As with NIH, training allocations in ADAMHA have declined to about 5 percent of research funds in 1988. Whereas NIH training obligations have declined about 17 percent in constant dollars, ADAMHA obligations for research training have been reduced by more than half since 1977 (Figure 5-8). There also has been a concomitant decline in the number of training positions, falling from 1,800 in 1977 to a low of 1,100 in 1986. The number of positions rebounded slightly, to nearly 1,300, in 1988 (Figure 5-9).

Training funds from NIH and ADAMHA are awarded through competitively reviewed institutional training grants or individual fellowship awards. About 85 percent of NIH-sponsored training appointments are supported on NRSA training grants awarded to institutions for either predoctoral (50 percent) or postdoctoral (35 percent) training.[27] Of the remaining training funds, 13 to 14 percent are awarded through NRSA individual postdoctoral fellowship awards, and slightly less than 2 percent are allocated to individual predoctoral fellowships. About 55 percent of the predoctoral training positions are awarded through the NIGMS followed distantly by NCI with

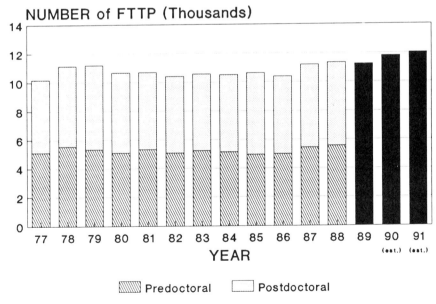

FIGURE 5-7   Number of full-time training positions (FTTPs) sponsored by the NIH from 1977 to 1991. (Appendix Table A-19)

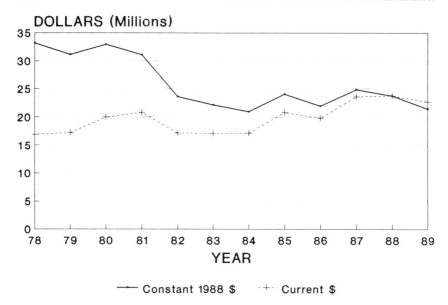

FIGURE 5-8   ADAMHA obligations for NRSA training. (Appendix Table A-20)

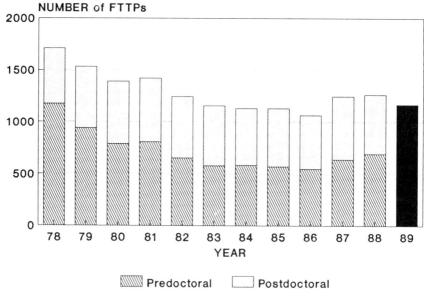

FIGURE 5-9   Number of full-time training positions (FTTPs) sponsored by ADAMHA from 1978 to 1989. (Appendix Table A-20)

10 percent of the predoctoral slots. NHLBI has the largest portion of postdoctoral positions—sponsoring about 20 percent of all NIH-supported postdoctorates.

Similar to NIH, about 87 percent of ADAMHA training funds are distributed through predoctoral and postdoctoral training grants, and only 13 percent support fellowship awards.[30] Currently, there is about equal distribution between predoctoral and postdoctoral support of full-time equivalent training positions in both NIH and ADAMHA. Whereas this ratio has been stable over the last decade for NIH, the cuts to research training in ADAMHA have affected only predoctoral positions, which have fallen from 1,178 to 694.[29,30] It should be noted that FTTPs totals are generally less than appointments because several short-term appointees can equal one FTTP.

The distribution between M.D. and Ph.D. postdoctoral training appointments has shifted slightly since 1980. In 1980 support was weighted more heavily toward Ph.D. postdoctorates, with 3,656 supported in comparison to 2,092 M.D. postdoctorates.[27] By 1987 the number of M.D. postdoctorates had increased to 2,532, thereby bringing support more in line with the 3,139 Ph.D. postdoctorates supported that year (Figure 5-10). Increased efforts to support more physician-scientists should increase the competitiveness of this group and enable them to win a larger share of investigator-initiated research project support.

The Medical Scientist Training Program (MSTP) sponsored by NIH is the largest national program for individuals pursuing joint M.D./Ph.D. degrees. This program is sponsored by NIGMS and has supported about 700 MSTP trainees annually throughout the 1980s.[27] Although the NIH funds programs in 28 medical schools, many more combined programs are supported in U.S. medical schools by private, state, and institutional funds. However, the committee was not able to determine the size of these commitments.[23]

The NSF Survey of Graduate Science and Engineering Students and Postdoctorates reports that large numbers of students are supported by teaching assistantships and a smaller but still significant number are supported on research grants.[13] Unfortunately, graduate students and postdoctoral fellows supported on research project grants from NIH and ADAMHA are not identified in the NIH database and the magnitude of this support, therefore, is difficult to ascertain. However, data from the Survey of Graduate Science and Engineering Students and Postdoctorates conducted by the NSF indicates a growing trend toward supporting trainees as research assistants on NIH research grants. The recent NRC report, *Biomedical and Behavioral Research Scientists: Their Training and Supply*, estimates that NIH supported research assistantships have grown from 2,673 in 1979 to 4,426 in 1987.

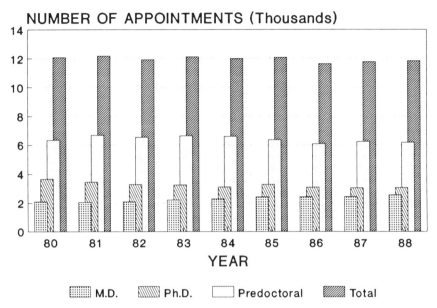

FIGURE 5-10   Number of trainee appointments in NIH sponsored training programs by academic level from 1980 to 1988. (Appendix Table A-21)

The MARC program administered by NIH attempts to address the problem of underparticipation by minority groups in the health sciences at both the undergraduate and graduate levels of training. Since 1982, NIH has supported about 400 MARC undergraduate training positions annually.[27] However, NIH support for MARC NRSA faculty fellowships has been dismal. In 1980 NIH supported only 36 of these faculty fellowships, and the number declined steadily to 18 in 1987. The committee believes that although this program offers the potential for recruiting individuals in minority groups into the health sciences, limited data do not allow a thorough program evaluation.

Other Support Mechanisms

By all measures, the private sector is increasing its commitment to training health scientists as well. According to one estimate, more than $17 million were invested in training by private foundations and voluntary health agencies. Contributions made at the undergraduate level generally provide support for curriculum development and improving the undergraduate teaching environment. For example, the Howard Hughes Medical Institute (HHMI) has initiated a series of grants programs to strengthen undergraduate science education and research in private undergraduate colleges and research universities with undergraduate colleges.[31] The goal of this program is to increase the number of students, especially minorities and women, pursuing careers in the biomedical sciences. In 1988 HHMI awarded $30.4 million to 44 colleges, including 10 historically black colleges. In the second year of the program the Institute expanded this initiative with $61 million awarded to colleges affiliated with research universities and other doctorate-granting institutions. Voluntary health agencies generally sponsor research fellowships or career development awards for postdoctoral training in their respective area of interest (e.g., cancer, heart disease, arthritis). Other programs target specific groups like the Robert Wood Johnson program to encourage underrepresented minorities to pursue careers in the health sciences including biomedical research.[32]

The committee believes that an increasing number of postdoctoral fellows are being supported by industrial sponsors. Favorable tax policy that has stimulated growing levels of investment in research and development may be responsible for this growing trend. Postdoctorates may be sponsored directly by the pharmaceutical or biotechnology industries to work in industrial R&D laboratories or, in some instances, in academic settings. It is unlikely that industry will invest significant amounts of funds at the undergraduate or predoctoral levels of training without more assurances that these trainees will be employed by their firms. Like foundations, corporate contributions for undergraduate and predoctoral education and training most likely will be used for curriculum development and updating the teaching environment. However, no centralized data base is available to determine either the magnitude of industry and private nonprofit support or the number of individuals supported. Clearly, the private sector can play a very significant role in training future health scientists, but the committee believes it simply cannot replace federal funding for research training.

SUMMARY AND CONCLUSIONS

The committee emphasizes that the single most critical long-term investment in the U.S. health sciences research enterprise is the sustained development of well-trained, creative scientists. Future progress toward improving health will continue only if efforts are sustained by talented individuals on all fronts to ensure a balanced attack on disease processes and exploration of all means of disease prevention. The emergence of an unexpected health crisis such as AIDS emphasizes the importance of trained scientific personnel who can be redirected quickly as needed. Successful handling of future epidemics will require a strong health sciences research system, particularly trained researchers.

Demographic data indicate that later this decade there will be increasing attrition of scientists trained in the 1950s and 1960s. Removing mandatory retirement ages may reduce some attrition due to retirements, but the effects will not be measurable until many years later. Employment growth in the private sector over the past decade has exceeded that in academia twofold. If this trend continues, competition for scientific talent between academia and industry will intensify.

Thus, evidence is mounting that the supply of health sciences researchers will be grossly inadequate to meet estimated demands by the end of this decade. These work-force trends will slow advances in the health sciences if they are not offset with careful planning and allocation of resources. In order to develop a highly qualified population of health scientists for the twenty-first century, the committee believes that:

• at a minimum, steps must be taken now to maintain the pool of scientific intellect in our society by improving the quality of science education and training;

• efforts must focus on recruiting, training, and retaining the most promising and talented individuals; and

• any new strategies should include programs targeted at increasing the numbers of scientists from underrepresented groups as well as improving multidisciplinary and interdisciplinary training of scientists.

Coordinated efforts across the educational spectrum are needed to sustain a pool of qualified health science researchers and to continue the progress already made in improving both the health care and quality of life of the American people. The failure to recruit qualified candidates into the health sciences is due partly to declining levels of support in the NRSA predoctoral and postdoctoral training programs as well as to neglect across the entire educational spectrum. The committee also concluded that the number of trainees supported on research project grants has been growing. Indeed, this type of support closely links research training with research. However, the committee acknowledges that there are disadvantages to supporting training on research project grants as well. Research grants commonly do not provide tuition support for graduate students since they may be classified as technical assistants receiving salary. The committee believes that often times support for these positions are reduced or removed when study sections provide recommended funding levels. Also, supporting trainees on research grants obligates trainees to perform established research protocols in order to ensure research productivity for the principal investigator(s) rather than acquiring a broad philosophical background for asking pertinent scientific questions. Policies therefore must be developed to address the needs of ongoing research as well as those ensuring the long-term vitality of the health sciences enterprise.

The committee is convinced that allocation policies in recent years emphasizing research project support have underemphasized the commitment for broad training experiences. Resource allocation policies should foster the development of highly qualified health researchers and should provide the opportunity for support throughout their careers. These policies should focus on the long-term goals of the research enterprise rather than short-term corrections. Academia, government, and industry must play cooperative roles in developing and pursuing effective strategies for enhancing and renewing the nation's health sciences talent base. Furthermore, allocation policies for training must prepare the nation for achieving its long-term research goals rather than merely making short-range adjustments to meet current needs.

REFERENCES

1. U.S. Congress; Office of Technology Assessment. 1988. Educating Scientists and Engineers: Grade School to Grad School. OTA-SET-377. Washington, D.C.: U.S. Government Printing Office.
2. Educational Testing Service. 1988. National Assessment of Educational Progress: The Science Report Card: Elements of Risk and Recovery. Princeton, N.J.
3. Lapoint, A.E., N.A. Mead, and G.W. Phillips. 1989. A World of Differences: An International Assessment of Mathematics and Science. Princeton, N.J.: Educational Testing Service.
4. National Research Council. 1989. Everybody Counts: A Report to the Nation on the Future of Mathematics Education. Washington, D.C.: National Academy Press.
5. Western Interstate Commission for Higher Education. 1988. High School Graduates: Projections by State, 1986 to 2004. Boulder, CO.
6. U.S. Congress; Office of Technology Assessment. 1985. Demographic Trends and the Scientific and Engineering Workforce. OTA-TM-SET-35. Washington, D.C.: U.S. Government Printing Office.
7. U.S. Department of Education, Office of Educational Research and Improvement. 1989. The Condition of Education, 1989: Postsecondary Education. Volume 2. CS 89-651. Washington, D.C.: National Center for Education Statistics.
8. National Academy of Sciences: The Government-University-Industry Research Roundtable. 1987. Nurturing Science and Engineering Talent: A Discussion Paper. Washington, D.C.: National Academy Press.
9. Abelson, P.H. 1989. Congressional fellowships for science. Science 243(4899):1649.
10. U.S. Department of Commerce: Bureau of the Census. Projections of the Population of the United States by Age, Sex, and Race, 1983 to 2080. Current Population Reports Series P-25, No. 925. Washington, D.C.
11. National Research Council. 1987. Minorities: Their Underrepresentation and Career Differentials in Science and Engineering (Proceedings of a Workshop). Washington, D.C.: National Academy Press.
12. Institute of Medicine. 1985. Minority Access to Research Careers: An Evaluation of the Honors Undergraduate Research Training Program. Washington, D.C.: National Academy Press.
13. NSF Science and Engineering Education Sector Studies Group. 1988. Selected Data on Graduate Science/Engineering Students and Postdoctorates, Fall 1987. Washington, D.C.: National Science Foundation.
14. National Science Foundation. 1988. Doctoral Scientists and Engineers: A Decade of Change. NSF 88-302. Washington, D.C.

15. National Research Council. 1989. Summary Report 1987, Doctorate Recipients from United States Universities. Washington, D.C.: National Academy Press.
16. National Research Council. 1987. Women: Their Underrepresentation and Career Differentials in Science and Engineering (Proceedings of a Workshop). Washington, D.C.: National Academy Press.
17. National Science Foundation. 1988. Characteristics of Doctoral Scientists and Engineers in the United States: 1987. NSF 88-331. Washington, D.C.
18. NSF Division of Policy Research and Analysis. 1989. Future Scarcities of Scientists and Engineers: Problems and Solutions. Washington, D.C.: National Science Foundation. (Working draft; April 25, 1989.)
19. National Research Council. 1989. Biomedical and Behavioral Research Scientists: Their Training and Supply. Washington, D.C.: National Academy Press.
20. Tuckman, H., S. Coyle, and Y. Bae. 1990. On Time to the Doctorate: A Study of the Increased Time to Complete Doctorates in Science and Engineering. Washington, D.C.: National Academy Press.
21. American Medical Association. 1987. Physician Characteristics and Distribution in the U.S. Chicago.
22. Jonas, H.S., and S.I. Etzel. 1988. Undergraduate medical education. JAMA 260(8):1063-1071.
23. Jonas, H.S., S.I. Etzel, and B. Barzansky. 1989. Undergraduate medical education. JAMA 262(8):1011-1019.
24. Institute of Medicine. 1988. Resources for Clinical Investigation. Washington, D.C.: National Academy Press.
25. National Science Foundation. 1987. Report on Funding Trends and Balance of Activities: National Science Foundation 1951-1988. NSF 88-3. Washington, D.C.
26. Institute of Medicine. 1985. Personnel Needs and Training for Biomedical and Behavioral Research. Washington, D.C.: National Academy Press.
27. U.S. Department of Health and Human Services. 1989. NIH Data Book 1989. National Institutes of Health Publication No. 90-1261. Bethesda, Md.
28. Moskowitz, Jay; Associate Director for Science Policy and Legislation, National Institutes of Health. 1989. Presentation at AAAS Symposia on Research and Development in the FY 1990 Federal Budget. Washington, D.C. April 1989.
29. Alcohol, Drug Abuse and Mental Health Administration. 1988. ADAMHA Data Source Book, FY 1987. Program Analysis Report No. 88-12. Washington, D.C.: U.S. Department of Health and Human Services.
30. Alcohol, Drug Abuse and Mental Health Administration. 1989. ADAMHA NRSA Research Training Tables, FY 1988. Program Analysis Report No. 89-15. Washington, D.C.: U.S. Department of Health and Human Services.
31. The Howard Hughes Medical Institute. 1987. Annual Report for 1987. Bethesda, Md.
32. The Robert Wood Johnson Foundation. 1987. Special Report: The Foundation's Minority Medical Training Programs. Number 1. Princeton, NJ.

6
Restoring the Physical Infrastructure for Health Sciences Research

The human element is critical to the conception and development of ideas, and the physical infrastructure for our scientific work force is vitally important as well. Over the past four decades, scientific knowledge has been expanding at an exponential rate. In order for this creativity to continue to flourish in the nation's research institutions, both within and outside of government, the scientist's physical environment must be conducive to high levels of scientific achievement. The laboratory buildings and libraries at research institutions house the essential tools that researchers need for scientific creativity to flourish. The scientific equipment and apparatus in those buildings, as well as the knowledge recorded and stored in the libraries, form the basis for the discovery of new knowledge.

According to various evidence, including surveys, interviews with scientists and administrators, and legislative testimony, laboratory facilities and equipment are becoming obsolete at an alarming pace, and the deteriorating condition of the physical research infrastructure limits the quality and quantity of research that can be carried out. The committee also emphasizes that unsuitable facilities will not only hamper research performance, but that unsuitable facilities will be a suboptimal training environment as well. Without adequate attention to facilities and equipment, the U.S. scientific work force will be seriously disadvantaged in its competition with the European and Japanese work forces.

The condition of physical structures has to be evaluated accurately, and laboratory equipment must be given equal attention. Advancing technology is encouraging the development of both more advanced equipment for old techniques as well as promoting newly designed equipment for new avenues of research. Although state-of-the-art tools may not be necessary to perform all laboratory tasks, increasing efficiency and accuracy by use of technologically advanced equipment inevitably will speed discovery and application of research results. Also, trainees need sufficient exposure to advanced technologies and equipment to be able to pose relevant research questions that will expand our medical knowledge base.

Federal regulations have elevated standards that render the present condition of many facilities no longer acceptable. Safety of laboratory personnel requires installation of certain costly equipment, such as improved fume hoods. Regulations on handling and disposal of radioactive and biohazardous wastes are becoming increasingly stringent, forcing a rise in overhead costs. These changes are most evident with the recent expansion of AIDS research, which requires highly specialized containment facilities for the study of the human immunodeficiency virus (HIV). Furthermore, there are increasing demands on utilities as equipment becomes more advanced and the electrical and plumbing systems needed to operate them properly must be up to date. Also, most new instrumentation requires climate-controlled environments in order to function properly. Changes in regulations and guidelines to protect animal welfare also add to the costs of performing research by forcing research institutions to modify buildings to meet changing caging and handling requirements.

Adverse conditions of the infrastructure may interfere directly with the ability to perform research or indirectly may discourage talented individuals from pursuing active research careers. Congress recognizes that research is hampered by aging and obsolete research facilities and instrumentation, and it admits that federal support for the construction of health sciences research facilities is one of the most complicated issues facing Congress.[1] Estimates of needs vary because of differences in definitions, sampling techniques, and time periods.

The National Institutes of Health (NIH) and the National Science Foundation (NSF) construction programs in the 1950s and 1960s greatly expanded the physical infrastructure for all scientific research—health sciences included. This period of expansion encouraged talented candidates to pursue careers in the sciences by providing the expectation of growth in research funding and adequate facilities and equipment to allow their ideas and creativity to flourish. Clearly, it would be impossible to build or renovate all health research facilities in order to make every institution a first tier research organization. However, it would not be sound policy to allow these institutions to crumble. According to the author of a recent article, "the government should decide how much science it is willing to pay for, but the long-run health of science will be jeopardized if uninformed and inconsistent policies result in too much money being put into current operational support and too little into facilities investment."[2]

This chapter reviews both the past and present federal programs for facilities construction and support for equipment as well as private sector contributions. The discussion focuses on the adequacy and suitability of existing research space and equipment and the financing mechanisms currently employed to build, renovate, and equip research facilities.

ADEQUACY AND SUITABILITY OF RESEARCH SPACE

The physical infrastructure for health sciences research in the United States includes facilities associated with the following institutions: colleges and universities, private independent research organizations, industry, and government laboratories. Most of the data available on biomedical research facilities and equipment concern the condition of college and university laboratories, although a survey that included nonfederal, nonprofit research facilities was conducted by NSF and NIH in 1988.[3,4] The committee is not aware of any data concerning the amount and adequacy of research space in industry.

The 1988 NSF/NIH survey reported that there was an estimated 52 million net assignable square feet (NASF) of biomedical research space at all institutions performing health research in the United States (Figure 6-1).[3] Forty-four million NASF (84 percent) of this space was located in academic institutions. The remaining 8 million NASF (16 percent) was distributed equally between independent research organizations and hospitals. Of the 44 million academic NASF, about 43 million NASF were located in doctorate-granting institutions and nearly half (21 million NASF) was in the top 50 research and development (R&D) institutions. Also, about two-thirds of all academic biomedical research facilities were located in public institutions. This distribution among the various types of public and private institutions has implications for the funding mechanisms available for construction and renovation.

In the same survey institutions were asked to rate the adequacy of their biomedical research facilities in the following categories: (1) adequate, (2) generally adequate, (3) inadequate, (4) nonexistent but needed, and (5) inapplicable or not needed. About half of the academic institutions rated their space as inadequate to support the needs of the research in the biological and medical disciplines (Figure 6-2). Medical schools had a slightly higher percentage (45 to 51 percent) of adequate space than did colleges and universities (37 to 46 percent). Academic institutions reported that 50 to 54 percent of their medical science research space and 45 to 46 percent of their biological science space generally was adequate. Very few academic

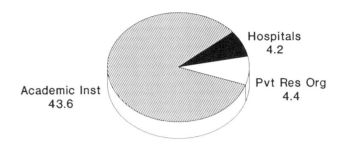

Millions of Net Assignable Square
Feet (NASF) for Biomedical Research

FIGURE 6-1   Distribution of U.S. biomedical research space.[3]

institutions (0 to 13 percent) reported that their space was able to support all of the needs of the research in these disciplines. Hospitals ranked their space much the same as the academic institutions, with nearly 45 percent of the space categorized as inadequate—the remainder being adequate or generally adequate. Independent research organizations reported a much higher percentage of adequate or generally sufficient space for research in the biological and medical sciences than did academic institutions, with 60 to 75 percent of the organizations rating the space in these two categories.

The physical condition of research facilities is related directly to the age of the structure. In 1986 the NSF reported that more than half (56.8 percent) of academic research facilities (all fields) were built prior to 1970, with about a quarter (26.5 percent) built or renovated before 1960.[5] Only 18 percent of research facilities were built or renovated between 1980 and 1986. Whereas these data are for research facilities in all fields, data from 71 institutions with medical schools demonstrate the same general trend.[5]

The 1988 NSF/NIH survey queried those same institutions on the suitability of existing research space for performing biomedical research. Only about one-quarter of the space for medical research at academic institutions was categorized as suitable for the most sophisticated research (Figure 6-3).[3] Whereas 35 to 41 percent of this space was categorized as adequate for most uses, one-quarter of the space required some repair or renovation, and 15 percent needed major repair or renovation. The condition of biomedical research space at research organizations generally was satisfactory, with nearly four-fifths of the space categorized as adequate for most uses or suitable for the most sophisticated research. However, 12 to 14 percent of the space in these institutions needed limited repair or renovation, and 10 to 13 percent required major work (Figure 6-3). Whereas hospitals reported that nearly half of their space for medical

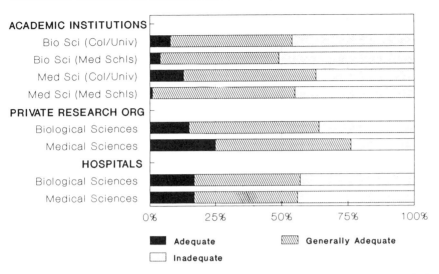

FIGURE 6-2 Adequacy of the amount of research space for biological and biomedical sciences.[3]

sciences was suitable for sophisticated research, about 20 percent required limited or major repairs. The suitability of space for the biological sciences in hospitals was rated as slightly worse.

Construction and Renovation Investment

It takes an average of 150 to 300 square feet of laboratory space to house an individual laboratory worker and his or her associated equipment.[3] Thus, a research group consisting of a director and 8 to 10 coworkers may require 2000 square feet or more. Large multidisciplinary teams may require as much as 10,000 square feet. The construction of laboratories that provide safe, proper space is estimated to cost more than $300 per square foot, and extensive renovation can be equally costly.[3]

The NIH reported that of the 16.7 million NASF of biomedical research space in need of repair and renovation at academic institutions, work on only 5.1 million NASF would be done in 1988 and 1989.[3] Thus, renovation and repair on the remaining 11.6 million NASF of space would be deferred. NIH estimated that the costs for planned renovation and repair would be $422 million, compared to a deferred amount of $920 million. Therefore, for every $1.00 of planned renovation and repair for 1988 and 1989, institutions were deferring an average of $2.18 of needed repair and renovations.

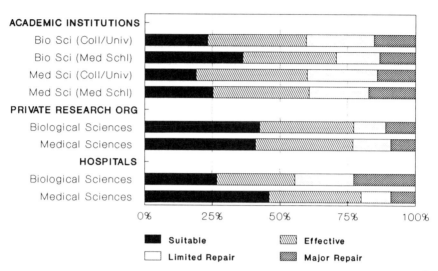

FIGURE 6-3   Current condition of research facilities in the biological and medical sciences.[3]

Variances in deferral ratios existed among the types of academic institutions (doctorate granting, medical schools, colleges, and universities) in the survey. Colleges and universities reported the largest deferral ratios— nearly $3.03 for every dollar planned for repair and renovation, which was twice the ratio of medical schools ($1.53) (Table 6-1). Of the nearly 2.2 million NASF of biomedical research space located in hospitals and research organizations needing repair and renovation, only 1.1 million was slated for repair and renovation in 1988 and 1989. The deferral ratio for hospitals was $0.52, whereas research organizations were deferring $1.53 for every $1.00 of planned repair and renovation.

Institutions also reported in the NSF/NIH survey that new construction was being deferred. Although "construction" may imply that these projects are for expansion of the current research plant, this may not be entirely true. Some new construction is planned to replace existing research space. That is, an out-dated facility may be demolished and replaced with a new facility. Although not increasing the NASF of research space of the institution, these new facilities will meet new building codes and provide a more suitable environment for advanced research.

According to the NSF/NIH survey, institutions reported actual and planned construction (renovation, replacement, and expansion) of biomedical research facilities totaling about $3.2 billion, with $2.7 billion at academic institutions, $0.2 billion at research organizations, and $0.3 billion at

TABLE 6-1 Comparison of Needed vs. Planned Repair/Renovation of Biomedical Research Facilities, by Institution Type, 1988-1989

	Repair/Renovation (R&R) Needs and Plans					
	Existing R&R Space (NASF in thousands)^a		Total Cost of^b (dollars in millions)			Ratio of Deferred: Planned R&R
Institution Type and Control	Needing R&R as of 1988	Planning R&R for 1988 & 89	All Needed R&R	All Planned R&R	Difference (deferred R&R)	
Academic institutions						
Total	16,700	5,120	1,342	422	920	2.18:1.00
Doctorate-granting						
Total	16,200	5,070	1,302	419	883	2.11:1.00
Top 50	8,300	2,640	667	258	408	1.59:1.00
Other	7,900	2,430	635	161	474	2.94:1.00
Non-doctorate-granting	400	50	32	3	29	9.67:1.00
Colleges and universities	8,900	2,410	715	177	538	3.03:1.00
Medical schools	7,700	2,710	619	245	374	1.53:1.00
Research organizations	1,001	622	101	40	61	1.53:1.00
Hospitals	1,166	497	117	77	40	0.42:1.00

^aNet assignable square feet.
^bAcademic estimates use $80.35 per square foot as the unit cost of repair and renovation. This rate was calculated by dividing the total cost of all planned R&R in 1988 or 1989 by the total NASF of planned R&R. Estimates for research organizations and hospitals use $100.68 square foot based on the unit cost of their repair/renovation projects.

SOURCE: U.S. Department of Health and Human Services; Public Health Service. 1988. The Status of Biomedical Research Facilities: 1988. Bethesda, Md.: National Institutes of Health.

independent hospitals. About $1.1 billion of the total investment was for projects initiated in 1986 and 1987. In 1988 and 1989 institutions planned a substantial increase in new facilities projects—about $2.1 billion.[3]

The NIH estimated that if all types of research institutions were to initiate construction to meet the needs of inadequate space (expansion construction only) in the biomedical sciences (and assuming the costs were the same per institution), $3.1 billion would be needed in 1988 and 1989. However, these research institutions planned construction of only $1.2 billion, creating a $1.9 billion shortfall for 1988 and 1989. Therefore, for every $1.00 in planned 1988 and 1989 construction, $1.63 was being deferred in needed but not planned construction.[3]

Again, there were large variances among the deferral ratios of the different types of institutions. Research organizations were deferring as much as $7.71 for every $1.00 of planned new construction in meeting the needs for the biomedical sciences (Table 6-2). Likewise, hospitals reported that they were deferring an average of $5.32 for every dollar spent on new construction in the biomedical sciences.

ADEQUACY AND SUITABILITY OF RESEARCH EQUIPMENT

Although it may be true that many pioneering discoveries in the health sciences were made by very simple means, scientists lacking access to proper instrumentation are limited in designing their experiments and collecting data, or they may be forced to turn away from some of the important problems of their discipline. A 1985 NIH study of 42 U.S. universities and 24 medical schools with the largest amounts of R&D funding collected information about instrumentation costs, age, condition, use, and so on.[6] More recently, NSF conducted a survey of academic research instrumentation in selected science and engineering fields, including the biological sciences in universities and medical schools.[7] These survey data, while appearing anecdotal, are the most accurate information available on the adequacy of research instrumentation for the health sciences.

The 1985 NIH survey, which queried the heads of 367 biological and medical science departments, provided some insight into the condition and needs of instrumentation in the health sciences.[6] Fifty-eight percent of the respondents indicated that critical scientific experiments could not be conducted because equipment was lacking. Although this response was more frequent in the biological sciences overall, 41 percent of the departments in medicine identified equipment shortages as a serious problem. Only 16 percent of the departments rated their equipment stocks as excellent for tenured faculty (15 percent for nontenured faculty). Between 50 and 60 percent of the respondents indicated that their equipment stocks were adequate, and nearly a third rated their equipment insufficient. These data

TABLE 6-2 Comparison of Needed vs. Planned Construction of Biomedical Research Facilities, 1988-1989 (dollars in millions)

Disciplines	Institutions with both Insufficient Space and Plans for New Construction		All Institutions with Insufficient Research Space[b]		Cost Difference (deferred construction)	Ratio of Deferred: Planned Construction
	Number of Institutions	Cost of Planned Construction	Number of Institutions	Cost of Needed Construction[c]		
Academic Institutions						
Total	—[a]	$1,195	—	$3,140	$1,945	$1.63:1.00
Biological sciences	61	400	228	1,203	803	2.01:1.00
Medical sciences	41	795	113	1,937	1,142	1.44:1.00
Research organizations						
Total	—	28	—	244	216	7.71:1.00
Biological sciences	5	12	45	108	96	8.00:1.00
Medical sciences	2	16	17	136	120	7.50:1.00
Hospitals						
Total	—	109	—	516	407	3.73:1.00
Biological sciences	3	87	13	377	290	3.33:1.00
Medical sciences	23	22	145	139	117	5.32:1.00

[a]Data not available.

[b]Insufficient space includes institutions reporting their current research space in the discipline as inadequate in amount or as nonexistent, but needed. Plans for new construction refers to plans to begin construction of new research space in the discipline in 1988 or 1989.

[c]Estimates were derived by multiplying per institution construction costs (as reported by institutions that plan construction in the discipline in 1988 or 1989) by the number of institutions reporting insufficient current space. To account for academic institution size differences, estimates were computed separately by institution type within discipline.

SOURCE: U.S. Department of Health and Human Services; Public Health Service. 1988. The Status of Biomedical Research Facilities: 1988. Bethesda, Md.: National Institutes of Health.

were collected in 1983, but the more recent data collected by NSF in 1986 showed no apparent change in response to similar questions.[7] In 1985 and 1986, 32 percent and 24 percent of department heads of the biological sciences in universities and medical schools, respectively, described their equipment as inadequate for pursuing their primary research interests. The working condition of equipment is related directly to its age. The upper limit for equipment to remain state of the art is estimated to be 5 years, with diminishing usability starting as early as the first year following purchase.[6] For instance, the median age of all 1985 and 1986 systems classified as state of the art by the principal user was only 2 years.[7] Technological advancement is one primary reason that research instrumentation becomes obsolete at an increasingly rapid pace. Thus, older equipment tends to be obsolete and frequently inoperable. The 1985 NIH survey reported that only 44 percent of the equipment in biological sciences and departments of medicine was less than 5 years old, about 29 percent was 6 to 10 years old, and the remaining 27 percent was more than 10 years old. This same survey revealed that only 18 percent of academic medical/biological instruments were classified as state of the art by respondents. About 65 percent of the instruments in active use were not classified as state of the art, and nearly 16 percent of equipment physically present in laboratories was not in use, owing either to mechanical disrepair or technological obsolescence. The survey showed also that only about half of the existing instrument systems were in excellent working condition.

The 1988 NSF study of academic research equipment in selected science and engineering fields reported that about one out of every four instrument systems in research use in 1982 and 1983 was no longer being used for research by 1985 and 1986.[7] Conversely, about two-fifths of all systems in research use in 1985 and 1986 had been acquired in the 3-year period since a 1982 and 1983 baseline study was conducted.

Maintenance and repair of existing equipment are additional problems for the users and host institutions. For every dollar spent to purchase equipment for the medical/biological sciences in 1983 (a total of $158.2 million), only 22.5¢ (a total of $35.7 million) was spent on maintenance and repair.[6] Moreover, maintenance and repair costs tend to increase after the instrument is over 5 years old.

SOURCES OF SUPPORT FOR FACILITIES AND EQUIPMENT

The traditional sources of capital for facilities and equipment are funds obtained from operations (tuition), gifts and foundation grants, government grants and contracts, and state and local government support. Other sources of funds for capital improvements may come from research partnerships or other arrangements with industry, debt financing, and the use of capital or operating leases. This diversification is necessary to help institutions adapt to changing economic environments by minimizing the effects of disruption from any one source. The mix of funding sources at any particular institution depends upon the type of institution (e.g., college, university, hospital or research organization, public or private sector).

Between 1986 and 1989 state and local governments were the primary sources of funding for new construction at universities and colleges, supplying about 46 percent ($1.8 billion) of all new construction money (Figure 6-4).[3] in contrast, 50 to 60 percent of new construction funds at medical schools, research institutions, and hospitals came from private monies or institutional funds. Tax-exempt bonds at all of these types of research organizations accounted for 17 to 30 percent of new construction funds. Facilities renovation or repair funds, however, largely were institutional monies, varying from 53 percent in medical schools to 72 percent at research organizations. About two-thirds of renovation and repair funds at universities and colleges came from institutional money and state and local government. During this period, the federal government provided very little support (0 to 8 percent) in the form of direct funds for all types of research organizations for facilities construction, repair, or renovation. An exception to this was federal support to historically black colleges and universities, which obtained more than 80 percent of their funding for construction and renovation projects from federal sources.[3]

The NIH has been the principal source of funding for medical and biological sciences equipment; for example, it funded nearly 38 percent of equipment in active use in 1983.[6] Equipment purchases are funded either directly, through research project grants, equipment grants, and block grants, or indirectly through indirect cost recovery mechanisms. Other federal agencies (including NSF) have funded about 12 percent of academic research instrumentation in the health sciences. Whereas the federal government funds nearly half of research equipment purchases, institutions provide the main portion (about 37 percent) of nonfederal funds for equipment. However, some institutional monies may have included indirect cost payments from research grants. Other sources of funds for equipment include state funds, private nonprofit foundations, and industry.[6]

State and Local Government

In recent years state and local governments have provided the largest proportion of funding for biomedical research facilities.[3] State governments invest in their colleges and universities to provide higher education for their citizens. The ability of individual states to support their institutions of higher education is related directly to their tax base. Investment decisions are made with respect to the state's industrial/agricultural profile,

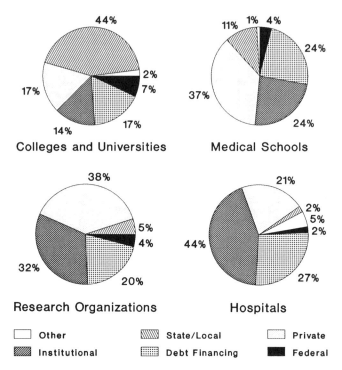

FIGURE 6-4   Source of facilities funding for the biological and medical sciences.[3]

labor force needs, and political or economic gains. Although states invest in facilities primarily to support education, they recognize that research is an integral part of the education process as well. Thus, states support research facilities construction projects to enhance higher education. States also have begun to look at investment in universities to improve economic development, as evidenced by the proliferation of state-supported biotechnology centers.

State support for equipment is estimated to be far smaller than the commitment to facilities construction and renovation. NIH estimates that state governments contribute only about 4 percent of the funds for biological and medical research equipment at academic institutions.[6] Since many states view research as a second priority in their institutions of higher education, fewer funds are available for equipment not used in classroom instruction.

Federal Grant Programs

Previous federal grant programs supported research facilities construction directly.[8] In federal construction programs Congress generally gives authority to NSF, NIH, the individual institutes of NIH, or another government agency or agencies to build research facilities. Funding decisions for money disbursed through these programs are based on competitively reviewed proposals. The criteria upon which these proposals are judged are determined by Congress and can include the following: (1) needs for expanding research capacity, (2) promotion of geographic distribution of research facilities, and (3) special programmatic needs. Previous NSF and NIH programs have required 50/50 matching funds from the recipient institution.

The first program to construct nonfederal research facilities began in 1948, through authority granted to the National Cancer Institute (NCI).[8] During the expansion of NIH in the 1950s, the physical infrastructure for scientific research had to be improved to pursue emerging scientific opportunities effectively. Then, in 1956, the Health Research Facilities Act (HRFA) authorized a Public Health Service (PHS) program to expand capacity, improve quality, and promote the equitable distribution of research in the health sciences. Grants made under this authority provided up to 50 percent of the costs for constructing, remodeling, altering, and equipping new or existing buildings for the health sciences. A primary condition for receipt of these funds was a 10-year commitment to use the designated facility for health sciences research.

Between 1956 and 1968 the HRFA program awarded 1,482 grants totaling $473 million to 407 institutions in all 50 states. Although this program required that only 50/50 matching funds be provided by the recipient institution, federal funds were matched with $632 million dollars (nearly 60 percent of construction costs) of institutional funds. Approximately 19 million net square feet of laboratory space—60 percent of the health-related research space constructed between 1958 and 1968—was built with the assistance of this program. Although this program was congressionally authorized until 1974, no funds were appropriated after fiscal year 1968. Unlike most NIH programs in which construction authority is targeted through institutes or disease programs, in the HRFA program the awards were made independent of these constraints.

Total NIH construction funds have been negligible over the past 10 years (Figure 6-5).[9] Only NCI, the National Eye Institute (NEI), and the National Heart, Lung and Blood Institute (NHLBI) have had construction authority in recent years. Construction obligations fell from $22 million in 1977 to $2 million in 1984 in constant dollars. Funding rebounded to $13 million in 1985, but it declined again to $9 million in 1986. In the 1988

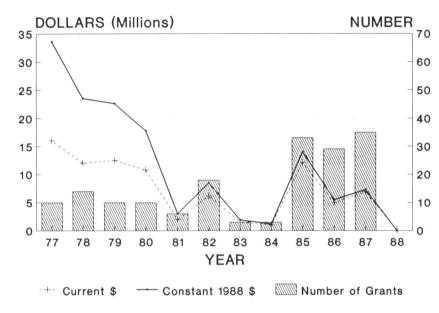

FIGURE 6-5   NIH allocations for extramural construction and number of grants awarded from 1977 to 1988.[9]

NIH reauthorization bill, $150 million of matching funds was proposed for construction—the most substantial increase in recent years. However, because the need for construction and renovation could not be verified adequately, these funds were not appropriated by Congress.[1]

Early construction authorities generally received separate appropriations, but recent authorities tend to be in direct competition with research funding. This has led to less use of these authorities by NHLBI and NEI and to declining construction support by NCI.[8] In fiscal years 1988 and 1989, no funds were requested under any of these construction authorities. However, $23.9 million was appropriated to the Division of Research Resources in fiscal year 1988 for AIDS-related construction.[10] The amount allocated in fiscal year 1989 was about $5 million.[11] A proposed $150 million facilities renewal fund was not approved for fiscal year 1990, although $14 million was taken from the institute budgets to fund a small program.

The NSF Science Facilities Program also contributed to the renovation and addition of large amounts of research space during the 1960s.[8] Whereas this program began by funding renovations and repair during the first couple of years, subsequent awards were made for building new and larger multidisciplinary structures as well as for purchasing stationary general purpose equipment. The program eventually was expanded beyond doctorate-granting institutions to those awarding masters degrees and to nonprofit institutions providing graduate training. This program granted 977 awards to 182 institutions. NSF estimated that awardees exceeded the 50 percent matching funds necessary for construction, supplying about 65 percent of the construction funds. Of the $188 million disbursed through this program, $500 million of new or renovated space and equipment was generated. Although the awards were made in all scientific disciplines, the life sciences received one-quarter of the funds and only 11 percent went to the behavioral sciences.

In 1960 the President's Science Advisory Committee issued a report entitled "Scientific Progress, the Universities, and the Federal Government," reaffirming the government's role in expanding the nation's research base.[8] After publication of this report, commonly known as the Seaborg Report; the NSF Science Development Grants Program became one of the agency's major programs between 1964 and 1972. Large grants were made to "second-tier" institutions to enable them to upgrade their research activities comprehensively over a 5-year period by providing funds to hire new faculty, support graduate students, and construct new facilities. Proposals for these grants were developed cooperatively between the institutions and NSF and were subject to peer review as well as an internal technical review. The program was divided into four sections, two of which provided considerable facilities funding. The University Sciences Development Program awarded $177 million to 31 institutions, and the Special Science Development Awards granted $44 million to 62 institutions. About 23 percent of these funds were used for facilities.[8]

Unlike direct support for facilities construction, equipment has been financed largely through funds from research project grants or shared instrument grants.[6] In 1966 11.7 percent of research project grant funds were used to purchase permanent laboratory equipment (Table 6-3). By the mid-1970s less than 5 percent of the funds awarded by NIH through research project grants as well as shared instrument programs were used for equipment. In 1984, the last year in the NIH survey, the percent of funds awarded by NIH for equipment was less than 4 percent of extramural awards, and has remained at this level through 1988. The committee was not able to determine the cause of this decline from the data available. Nevertheless, it is concerned that if this trend continues, scientists may not be able to conduct necessary research protocols in a high-quality manner on NIH grant awards.

Earmarking funds for universities, often referred to as pork barreling, has become commonplace in the 1980s. For instance, in fiscal year 1982 Congress earmarked about $3 million for projects on specific university campuses,[12] and by 1989 the total earmarking to universities had reached almost $300 million.[13] Whereas construction funds allocated to science agencies such as NIH and NSF are awarded to colleges and universities in

TABLE 6-3 Percent of NIH Research Project Grant Funds Allocated for Permanent Laboratory Equipment, Fiscal Years 1966-1988

Year	Percent	Year	Percent
1966	11.7	1978	4.4
1967	11.8	1979	4.6
1968	9.5	1980	3.8
1969	7.5	1981	3.3
1970	5.9	1982	3.2
1971	6.2	1983	3.4
1972	6.6	1984	3.7
1973	4.9	1985	4.1
1974	5.7	1986	3.7
1975	4.6	1987	4.0
1976	3.9	1988	3.9
1977	4.3		

SOURCES: U.S. Department of Health and Human Services; Public Health Service. 1985. Academic Research Equipment and Equipment Needs in the Biological and Medical Sciences. NIH Program Evaluation Report No. 85-2769. Bethesda, Md.

U.S. Department of Health and Human Services; Public Health Service. 1989. NIH Data Book Publication No. 90-1261. Bethesda, Md.: National Institutes of Health.

competitive programs, earmarking bypasses all scientific merit and technical review. The committee believes that the direct lobbying of congressional members by universities ultimately will benefit only a few institutions and not necessarily those with a definite need.

Indirect Cost Recovery

Indirect cost (IDC) recovery is a reimbursement mechanism used by institutions to recoup expenses already incurred. Although the federal government does not restrict the use of these funds, there are guidelines that outline reimbursable expenses. For instance, federal IDC funds cannot pay for the use of facilities originally financed with federal funds. Also, whereas indirect payments reimburse the institution for the original cost of the facility, institutions are not reimbursed for replacement costs.

Institutions receiving federal research funds negotiate individual IDC rates with the sponsoring agency.[14] Many foundations and some industrial sponsors set limits on IDCs allowable. Under current practice, IDCs are used largely for operations and maintenance of the research facilities and ancillary costs of doing research. There is a small percentage (2 percent) of IDC that can be used for depreciation of research facilities, assuming a 50-year life-span of buildings. This assumption may not reflect the life-span of research facilities accurately, for these facilities may become outdated in only 20 years.[15,16]

Use allowances, depreciation, and interest payments (since 1982) on debts for facilities used in sponsored research are allowable reimbursements to universities through IDC recovery. As larger portions of facilities construction money comes from nonfederal sources, this portion of IDCs is edging upwards and increasing the overall institutional rate.[17]

As the funds for construction grant programs came to an end in the late 1960s and early 1970s, the government shifted its policy to support facilities through IDC recovery to research institutions.[8] With additional emphasis on research projects in the 1980s, this policy has become ensconced as the primary means of federal support for facilities renewal. This allows investigators to apply for equipment funds freely, but little if any money is for research buildings except through IDC recovery.

The committee believes this policy of IDC recovery as the sole source of facilities renewal is fundamentally flawed. There is a direct relationship between the level of sponsored research activity and IDC reimbursement, which is part of the financial support package to institutions performing the research. The short duration of grant support, generally less than 4 years, contributes to the tendency of research institutions to meet short-term needs rather than the long-range planning necessary for science. Also, whereas the IDCs recovered by the top 50 institutions can be substantial, IDC recovery by second-tier institutions can do little for major construction needs at these institutions.

The Office of Management and Budget (OMB) Circular A-21, which regulates the recovery of IDCs related to federally sponsored research, was first written in the 1950s.[18] Ceilings were placed on institutions' IDC rates until 1966; therefore, associated research costs could not be recovered fully. Although the cap no longer exists, there is speculation that many institutions underreport IDCs to keep the overall costs of research low, thus helping their individual institutions remain competitive nationally. Also, as pressures mount to keep IDC categories down, many institutions may shift some of these costs to direct cost categories; thus, total awards will remain the same, but with larger percentages in the direct cost category. Also, the budget sheets of research grants, which include IDC rates and amounts, are available to study section members and may influence awards especially in times of extremely scarce research funds.

Debt Financing

Debt financing is used by academic institutions as one means of raising funds for capital improvements. Whereas debt financing by state institutions is controlled by state legislatures, private institutions use tax-exempt bonds to raise capital for facility improvements. Also, limits on debt financing through tax-exempt bonds are set by the federal government. The 1984 Tax Reform Act placed a state per capita limit on student loan issues and limited industrial development bond issues. Further restrictions were imposed by the 1986 Tax Reform Act, which limited institutional tax-exempt borrowing to $150 million.

For institutions to be able to use the bond market, they must be good credit risks. Credit evaluations of academic and research organizations are similar to that of corporations because they are judged on their estimated future earnings and past performance for repaying debt. The ability of faculty to get grants is not a major consideration in credit evaluations. Therefore, only well-established institutions with a good credit rating can use this financial instrument to fund facilities projects. It is estimated that only about 10 percent of the colleges and universities in the United States have effective access to the tax-exempt market.[8] Since there is an economy of scale in bond issues, institutions frequently combine various facilities (e.g., parking garages, dormitories, and laboratories) into one bond issue.

Tax-exempt bonds are particularly attractive financial instruments for private academic institutions, because these institutions can borrow facilities construction money at interest rates below the interest income levels received on their endowments. However, restrictions in the 1986 Tax Reform Act placed a $150 million limit on outstanding bond debt for private institutions. Nearly 27 percent of the medical schools are affiliated with institutions who have reached this limit, and another 10 percent are expected to do so within the next 2 years.[3] This severely limits these institutions' ability to undertake large construction projects, including modifying and expanding research space.

The federal government currently sponsors two programs to encourage loans to academic institutions for capital improvement. Congress authorized the Student Loan Marketing Association (nicknamed Sallie Mae), through the Higher Education Amendments of 1986, to lend funds for academic facilities construction. Seventy-five percent of these loans must be made to institutions with credit ratings below the third highest rating. The second program, the College Construction Loan Insurance Corporation (nicknamed Connie Lee), authorized by the Higher Education Amendments of 1986, established a program to guarantee, insure, or reinsure bonds and other debt instruments for academic facilities.[17]

Institutional Funds

In addition to federal, state, and local government support, institutions of higher education obtain revenues from tuition, philanthropy, endowment income, and revenues from sales and services. The proportions of support from these various sources have changed over the last decade, with government support declining and revenue from the other sources increasing.

Recent evidence of this is the skyrocketing costs of college tuition in both private and public institutions.[20]

The Government-University-Industry Research Roundtable (GUIRR) reports that almost 20 percent of facilities funds annually came from institutional monies in the years 1986 through 1989.[17] Publicly supported institutions devoted 15 percent of institutional funds for facilities, whereas these monies constituted 24 percent of the facilities funds expended at private institutions. Institutions also fund nearly as much research equipment in the biological and medical sciences as does the NIH: 37 and 38 percent, respectively.[6] Unrestricted institutional funds can be used as matching funds for government facilities and equipment grants. Escalating education costs, which have continued to outpace inflation, coupled with possible declining enrollments in the 1990s, inevitably will increase competition within institutions for distributing endowment earnings between educational and research needs.

Gifts and donations from philanthropies are other sources of funding for constructing and restoring facilities. Private institutions rely heavily on these sources to raise money for capital improvements: About 20 percent of the science and engineering facilities funding between 1986 and 1989 was provided through gifts and donations.[17] Unlike institutional funds, which are controlled by the institutional officers, donors often restrict the use of gifts and donations; therefore, institutions have less control over their use. Also, philanthropic giving is affected directly by tax law. Whereas the Tax Reform Act of 1986 has reduced the marginal tax rates, it treats gifts of appreciated property as a preference item and subjects them to the alternative minimum tax of 21 percent.[21] The effect of tax law changes on philanthropic giving has been studied by expert groups, and a clear conclusion on the result remains elusive.

Foundations and Voluntary Health Agencies

Foundations and voluntary health agencies support facilities through direct and indirect means. These organizations can contribute directly through specific facilities and equipment programs or indirectly through comprehensive curriculum development programs with allowances for facilities construction. For example, the Kresge Foundation Science Initiative is a matching funds grant program for scientific equipment and laboratories that provides foundation funds to colleges and universities to upgrade equipment.[22] Indirectly, these types of organizations support facilities through payment of overhead costs associated with grants to the facility. However, the committee believes that these organizations cap IDC rates, and, therefore, they do not pay the full costs for performing the research they sponsor.

Industrial Participation

Many corporations support their own R&D facilities, but the magnitude of this support is unknown. Industries have not been significant supporters of research facilities projects at academic institutions or independent research organizations. Rather, companies have preferred direct project or program funding in which they have greater leverage or control. It is believed that companies, like foundations, may tend to increase IDC recovery problems for universities by negotiating lower overhead rates than what federal sponsors pay.[23]

In recent years partnerships have spawned between industry and universities.[24] These arrangements are intended to provide mutual benefits to both parties without compromising the educational mission of the university. Although individual project support from industry generally does not provide full recovery of IDCs, the committee believes these larger partnerships sponsored by industry provide more reimbursement for facilities and administrative costs of performing the research than individual projects allow.

SUMMARY AND CONCLUSIONS

The committee concludes that aging research space and obsolete equipment are restricting the number and types of research projects that can be undertaken. Over the last decade there has been a plethora of studies on the condition of academic facilities, and there is general agreement within, as well as outside, the scientific community that many research laboratories on our campuses are in disrepair. The committee concludes that even after repeated studies, no long-term federal strategy exists to restore the physical infrastructure. There is no consensus on the need for expanded versus renovated facilities, the best mechanism for support, and the respective roles of the interested parties. Additionally, there is no way to coordinate the various independent contributors supporting facilities and equipment. Without a clear set of goals and a cohesive national policy, universities and other research institutions will be forced to continue seeking short-term solutions to their facilities' needs by obtaining earmarked appropriations from Congress.

At a minimum, the committee believes it is critical to maintain the current level of research effort as well as provide an optimal environment for training the next generation of health scientists. Meeting these objectives is becoming increasingly more difficult under the present condition of research facilities. It will be counterproductive to allow the existing facilities to slip into a further disrepair where scientists will no longer be able to investigate the frontiers of science. The committee could not conclude that all outmoded structures should be renovated; rather, those structures that can be updated should be, and the others should be demolished and rebuilt. The committee also believes that the decline in federal programs for research facility construction and equipment is partially responsible for deterioration of the nation's research laboratories. Federal support of facilities and equipment as a percentage of total federal health R&D expenditures has decreased drastically over the past two decades. Federal grant programs in the 1960s were very successful in expanding the nation's research capabilities, but several factors caused the NIH and NSF facilities programs to be eliminated in the early 1970s.

Except for some limited appropriations for AIDS research facilities, federal funds for health sciences research facilities have been negligible or nonexistent over the past 10 years. This comes at a time of escalating maintenance costs, increasing regulatory standards, and an explosion of scientific opportunities and technological sophistication. Although research institutions have been able to raise some money from other sources, a great deal of biomedical research renovation and money construction needs are being deferred.

Creative funding mechanisms will be required to fill the enormous need for new and renovated biomedical research facilities, now estimated to be in excess of $8 billion—more than three and one-half times the amount to be spent. Alternatives to the traditional forms of capital formation are beginning to reshape the way academia raises money for capital improvements. State and local governments are investing in academic facilities for education and garnering the economic advantages of providing a sound scientific base in the state. Although the private sector continues to make significant contributions to supporting the physical infrastructure of research, it cannot be expected to meet the total need. Partnerships with industry (although limited) may help fill these enormous gaps for research institutions but are sensitive arrangements to work out.

It seems that the policy options available are few. As IDCs increase, scientists claim that they consume scarce research resources. Institutional administrators claim that overhead rates are undercharged and that they have to find these resources to keep their institutions competitive. With large federal deficits looming in the immediate future, direct grant programs for revitalizing the physical infrastructure seem remote. Thus, it appears that we will be forced to recoup these costs through indirect means.

Despite these problems, the committee concluded that there is a crucial need to establish a national policy for renewal and expansion of the health sciences research infrastructure. The objectives of a comprehensive facilities plan should be twofold:

1. To maintain and restore the present physical infrastructure by improving the capabilities and efficiency of performing health sciences research.

2. To expand the physical infrastructure and therefore the nation's capacity to perform health sciences research.

Meeting these objectives will allow scientists to pursue new as well as existing opportunities in the health sciences in order to expand the boundaries of health sciences knowledge.

REFERENCES

1. U.S. House of Representatives. 1989. Report of the House of Representatives Appropriations Subcommittee for the Departments of Labor, Health and Human Services, and Education, and Related Agencies Appropriations Bill, 1989. Report No. 100-689. Washington, D.C.

2. Massey, W.F. 1989. Capital investment for the future of biomedical research: A university chief financial officer's view. Acad Med 64(1989):433-437.

3. U.S. Department of Health and Human Services; Public Health Service. 1988. The Status of Biomedical Research Facilities: 1988. Bethesda, Md.: National Institutes of Health.

4. National Science Foundation. 1988. Scientific and Engineering Research Facilities at Universities and Colleges. NSF 88-320. Washington, D.C.

5. National Science Foundation. 1986. Science and Engineering Research Facilities at Doctorate-Granting Institutions. Washington, D.C.

6. U.S. Department of Health and Human Services; Public Health Service. 1985. Academic Research Equipment and Equipment Needs in the Biological and Medical Sciences. NIH Program Evaluation Report No. 85-2769. Bethesda, Md.

7. National Science Foundation. 1988. Academic Research Equipment in Selected Science/Engineering Fields: 1982-82 to 1985-86. NSF SRS 88-D1. Washington, D.C.

8. U.S. House of Representatives. 1987. Brick and Mortar: A Summary and Analysis of Proposals to Meet Research Facilities Needs on College Campuses. Committee on Science, Space, and Technology; Subcommittee on Science, Research, and Technology; GPO Publication No. 77-341. Washington, D.C.

9. U.S. Department of Health and Human Services; Public Health Service. 1988. NIH Data Book, 1988. Publication No. 89-1261. Bethesda, Md.: National Institutes of Health.

10. NIH Budget Office.

11. U.S. Congress. 1988. Departments of Labor, Health and Human Services, and Education, and Related Agencies Appropriations Act, 1989. P.L. 100-436.

12. Panning pork. 1988. Science 242:1383.

13. Cordes, C. 1989. Colleges receive about $289-million in earmarked funds. The Chronicle of Higher Education. February 1, pp. A1 and A20.

14. Association of American Universities. 1988. Indirect Costs Associated with Federal Support on University Campuses: Some Suggestions for Change (Draft). AAU Ad Hoc Committee on the Indirect Costs to the Executive Committee of the AAU. Washington, D.C.

15. U.S. Department of Health and Human Services. 1988. Report of the Ad Hoc NIH Study Group on Extramural Biomedical Research Facilities Construction. Bethesda, Md.: National Institutes of Health.

16. U.S. Department of Health and Human Services. 1989. Report on Extramural Biomedical Research Facilities Construction. Office of the Secretary. Washington, D.C.

17. National Academy of Sciences; Government-University-Industry Research Roundtable. 1990. Perspectives on Financing Academic Research Facilities: A Resource for Policy Formulation. In Press.

18. Office of Management and Budget. 1979. Principles for Determining Costs Applicable to Grants, Contracts, and Other Agreements with Educational Institutions. OMB Circular A-21. Washington, D.C. (Revised February 1979.)

19. National Association of College and University Business Officers. 1988. Capital Formation Alternatives in Higher Education. NACUBO Capital Management Series. Washington, D.C.

20. The College Board. 1989. The College Cost Book, 1989-90. New York: College Board Publications.

21. Ginzberg, E., and A.B. Dutka. 1989. The Financing of Biomedical Research. Baltimore: The Johns Hopkins University Press.

22. The Kresge Foundation. 1987. Annual Report for 1987. Detroit.

23. National Academy of Sciences: Government-University-Industry Research Roundtable. 1986. Academic Research Facilities: Financing Strategies. Washington, D.C.: National Academy Press.

24. National Academy of Sciences; Government-University-Industry Research Roundtable. 1986. New Alliances and Partnerships in American Science and Engineering. Washington, D.C.: National Academy Press.

7

Policy Overview and Recommendations

SUPPORT FOR HEALTH SCIENCES RESEARCH

Since World War II, U.S. health science policy has led to an unquestionably successful health research enterprise. This growth and development has been nurtured by a unique mixture of research sponsors: the federal government, state governments, private foundations and voluntary health agencies, and corporations. This multifaceted support system has invested large amounts of resources into building an unequaled health research infrastructure. Such a diversified system of support has diminished the potential for centralized planning and has encouraged input from a wide range of views regarding the conduct of health sciences research ensuring that no one group could impose limitations on what ideas should be pursued or how the research should be conducted. In effect, this unique research system has preserved academic freedom and encouraged the creativity of health scientists allowing them to develop and test their hypotheses for improving our understanding of human disease processes. *The committee concluded that preserving this broad-based support system is essential to continue a vigorous U.S. health sciences research program.*

Opportunities in health sciences research appear to be growing almost exponentially. However, the number of excellent ideas far exceeds the available funding. In order to maintain the momentum for supporting the best science resources have to be allocated to the various components of the research enterprise. The committee emphasizes that the components of the research infrastructure are highly interrelated and dependent upon one another, and scientists will not be able to deliver optimum research results and train young investigators without adequate facilities and equipment. Likewise, overemphasis on increasing research space will be to no avail if the buildings are underutilized by scientists and mentors because of shortages of researchers and research funds. *The charge to this committee was to analyze the entire research infrastructure (people, projects, facilities, and equipment) in a holistic fashion and develop a coordinated set of policies to ensure balanced allocations to the components of the research system: people, projects, and facilities.*

Although the committee acknowledges that many of the previous accomplishments in the health sciences have been directly attributed to the magnitude of federal support for health research, the charge to the committee did not include justifying a basis for increasing congressional appropriations. Undoubtedly, this phase of the allocation process is critically important to the continued success of the health sciences research enterprise. Because of the overwhelming success of previous health research endeavors, new and heuristic research opportunities are emerging continuously. However, such opportunities easily could consume substantial increases in funding. Although this study does not address the process for increasing congressional appropriations, the committee acknowledges that the level of future research support from Congress will be related directly to the potential societal benefits of health research. The primary goal of this committee in developing a balanced allocation process was to preserve the creativity of the individual investigator—the most valuable asset to the research enterprise. *Beyond the role of the federal government, the committee believes that better inter-sectoral communication among the government, industry, and private nonprofit sponsors of health sciences research is necessary to meet this challenge.*

Patterns and Policies of Federal Health Sciences Support

Federal support for basic research has been based on the following five principles:

1. *Stable federal support* for research in order to undertake long-range programs.
2. *Peer review for evaluating scientific merit* of all research projects paid for by federal funds.
3. *Academically based scientific investigation.*
4. *Flexible scientific research management* policies left to individual scientists and their institutions.
5. *Accountability to the Congress, the President, and the American public.*

Although many changes have evolved in the way science is supported by the federal government, these general principles have stood the test of time. Many private and nonprofit sponsors of health research have adopted them as well.

Research Community Perceptions

The committee closely analyzed federal funding trends and policies for health sciences research over the past two decades. Additionally, the committee reviewed the limited data available on the contributions from other governmental sources, private foundations and voluntary health agencies, and corporate research sponsors. These analyses revealed a continuous commitment to the support of the health sciences research enterprise in terms of both absolute and relative dollars. Funding patterns through 1989 revealed that more investigators and projects are receiving federal support than ever before, with the highest total allocations since the system began. Furthermore, despite federal budget cuts in many nonhealth domestic programs throughout the past decade, health sciences research has continued to receive annual increases in appropriations through fiscal year 1990.

Regardless of these gains, there is a strong feeling within the scientific community that federal support for future health research is unstable and unpredictable. Much of the concern is based upon two often cited statistics: (1) the declining number of annual new and competing awards and (2) the decline in annual award rates (award rate = grants awarded/total approved applications). Adding to the confusion, NIH and ADAMHA recently have replaced the former system for awarding grants based upon raw priority scores with a more complex moving average percentile ranking system.

In the new percentiling system the raw priority scores assigned to grant applications in the current review cycle of a particular study section are percentiled with priority scores from the two previous review cycles. In effect, percentiling diminishes the variance of the priority scores assigned by a particular study section over three review cycles. Once the slate of grant applications is presented to the various institutes, the institutes determine a certain percentile threshold for proposals to be awarded. By selecting a percentile funding cut-off for awarding grants, the variance in priority scores among different study sections is normalized. Since its inception, however, the percentile cut-off generally has been misconstrued by the scientific community as the award rate. For example, institutes may be funding to the 12th or 13th percentile but this translates into a 24-25 percent award rate. Thus, the low percentile cut-off has led to a false impression of "declining" support for health sciences by NIH and ADAMHA.

Adding to this misperception are other less explicit policy changes and disturbances within the health research environment reflected in award rates. For example, the policy to lengthen grant awards, which has increased the average duration of research grants from 3.2 years to approximately 4 years, implies that about 25 percent fewer grants will need to be renewed each year to sustain the same overall annual number of research projects supported by NIH and ADAMHA. Since 1976, the number of grant applications submitted for peer review has continued to outpace the growth in appropriations. This dramatic growth in the number of investigator-initiated research project applications reflects, in part, a surge in research opportunities as well as the growing practice of applying for multiple grant awards.

Simultaneously, the approval rate for grant applications by study sections has risen steadily, from 70 percent in the mid 1970s to nearly 95 percent. As a result, the growth in applications, combined with the increasing approval rate, has driven down the award rate throughout the 1980s (Figure 4-8). Despite recent declines in annual new and competing awards, the total portfolio of NIH grant awards (competing plus noncompeting continuations) has grown every year from the early 1970s until 1988. Although the total number of awards supported by NIH dropped by 200 in 1989, from 20,867 to 20,681, and further to 20,316 in 1990, the NIH investment committed to research in real dollar amounts has continued to grow. The total number of awards is expected to increase slightly by nearly 125 in fiscal year 1991.

These policy changes have created substantial long-term pressures on the infrastructure of the research enterprise. Despite the overall long-term upward trend in research funding, these longer-term concerns became the primary motivation for this study. The committee has analyzed all of the available data pertaining to the overall level of support for research projects and has found no evidence to confirm the research community's perception of declining federal research support. To clarify these issues and to recommend corrections, the next section summarizes policy decisions, both implicit and explicit, that have contributed to the current anxieties within the research community.

A Brief Review of Past Policy Decisions for Resource Allocation

The First 20 Years: Balanced Growth in Research Support

Between 1950 and 1968 NIH underwent rapid growth. Federal policies combined with growing congressional appropriations fostered considerable flexibility for funding research, with support being provided for all four of the interdependent components of the research enterprise: (1) a well-trained pool of researchers, (2) modern facilities, (3) modern equipment, and (4) research project funding.

During this era, various mechanisms for supporting research were established in an effort to control disease and improve health. While investigator-initiated research and development (R&D) grants have been the cornerstone of NIH and ADAMHA extramural programs during the postwar expansion, other mechanisms for investigator-initiated research support have included program project grants, center grants, and, more recently, cooperative agreements. R&D contracts have been yet another mechanism for supporting research, although contracts commonly are not investigator initiated. There has also been a strong federal commitment to train researchers and to build research facilities.

Constrained Growth and Instability in the 1970s

"Stabilization" Policy. Slower budgetary growth in the 1970s along with a dramatic inflation rate reduced the buying power of research dollars. One result of these forces was the fluctuating number of annual new and competing grants awarded in the late 1970s. For example, between 1975 and 1976 the number of new and competing awards dropped from 4,700 to 3,500—a drop of nearly 25 percent—and then surged to 5,200 in 1978. These fluctuations led to uncertainty in the availability of ongoing support for health research. Consequently, the scientific community began to lose confidence in the future of federal research support.

In response to these concerns, Congress, NIH, and ADAMHA agreed to a policy that established a minimum number of new and competing research project grant applications to be funded annually. Beginning in fiscal year 1981 and ending in 1988, minimum numbers of new and competing awards were established between NIH/ADAMHA and the congressional appropriations committees. This decision, in turn, reflected an explicit NIH/ADAMHA policy that investigator-initiated research project grants were the highest priority for their current research programs and that maintaining a minimum level of new awards would stabilize the health research base. However, the Administration's budget requests for NIH and ADAMHA also had to conform to the Department of Health and Human Services (DHHS) budgets. DHHS budgets were, in turn, highly influenced by budget balancing in the Office of Management and Budget (OMB).

"Downward Negotiation" Policy. Despite added appropriations from congressional committees, the available funds were inadequate to fund fully the agreed upon number of awards. Thus, in order to comply, NIH and ADAMHA were forced into a policy of reducing ongoing research commitments (noncompeting continuing awards from previous years) as well as the

amounts paid to new and competing awards in what commonly is referred to as downward negotiation. This is a recent practice for reconciling NIH and ADAMHA research grant commitments to annual appropriations by making across-the-board reductions in all grant awards. Downward negotiation is a euphemism, since little if any negotiation actually occurs between the scientist and NIH or ADAMHA. Rather, these decisions concerning the overall proportions of the previously committed funds to be withheld in order to fund the required annual level of new and competing awards are made between NIH/ADAMHA and OMB. This policy has placed additional burdens on scientists, for they are expected to perform the proposed research with less than the recommended amount of funding.

The committee concluded that the stabilization policy was a sound strategy to protect the research base. However, the necessary appropriations to support fully the ongoing research obligations of NIH and ADAMHA were not provided. As a result, NIH and ADAMHA were forced to make arbitrary administrative cuts in all grant awards to be able to fund the mandated new and competing grants. While the overall grant portfolio grew, these cuts contributed to instability in the research project support system as well as to an imbalance among support for the other components of the research enterprise.

Further Constraints and Crises in the 1980s

"Extended Duration of Awards" Policy. Although NIH and ADAMHA were increasing the numbers of new and competing awards through the stabilization policy, the research community felt that the average 3-year award period for traditional research project grants (R01) was too short. Three-year awards do not allow for long-term research program planning, nor, in many cases, do they allow scientists sufficient time to achieve research goals. Additionally, these shorter-duration awards require too much emphasis on grant writing and administrative details.

As competition intensified throughout the 1980s, the number of grant applications with very high priority scores increased. Nevertheless, despite high priority scores, any given ongoing research project faced termination if its score in competitive renewal fell just below the pay line. With interrupted funding, individual scientists felt they would be forced to reduce staff below critical levels, and although amended applications might ultimately restore funding to the program, the research team may by then have been disbanded. As a consequence of these fears, multiple grant applications, with renewals in alternate years, were seen by many scientists as a means of providing continuity of funding for their research programs.

To address these concerns, NIH and ADAMHA instituted a policy to increase the length of grant awards gradually. The intended results of increasing award periods were to provide more stability in research activities and scientists' careers and, possibly, to discourage the number of multiple grant applications by individual investigators. Additionally, longer award periods were viewed as a means to reduce the administrative workload for NIH and ADAMHA study sections by reducing the number of competitive renewal applications processed each year.

Although increasing grant duration does have a stabilizing effect on research careers, it also obligates NIH and ADAMHA appropriations further into the future. This policy of lengthening award periods, coupled with the phenomenon of increasing average award size, reduces the funds available for meeting annual targets of new and competing grant awards. *Despite these problems, the committee believes it is no longer justifiable to sacrifice the stability of support for productive scientists simply to maintain a given annual quota of grant awards. To this end, the committee supports this NIH and ADAMHA policy to extend award periods, even if it reduces the number of new and competing awards in any single year. Despite the consequence of a sharp reduction in new and competing awards in a correction year, the system will once again attain a balance in the out years.*

Peer Review Process and Allocation Policy

The committee also heard testimony from the scientific community about the effectiveness of the peer review process for evaluating grant proposals. As the proportion of approved proposals receiving funds has declined over the past decade, many scientists believe that the peer review process has favored the "old boy network" of mid to late career investigators who have been receiving continuous research support at the expense of young creative scientists just entering the competitive grant system. While there are data demonstrating that the average age of principal investigators is increasing, there is no evidence that these older scientists are less creative or that their grant applications are less meritorious.

It is commonly believed that many scientists are reluctant to submit innovative or high-risk proposals because the review panels may be averse to recommending funding for less conventional research. Prevention and nutrition research are examples of proposals that may not fair well in the present structure of peer review for various reasons. Because of the confidentiality of unfunded research grant proposals, no data exist on the number of "novel" proposals not awarded. However, the committee acknowledges that a closer examination of the peer review system and its role in determining the effectiveness and efficiency of expended research funds may be warranted.

Conclusions on Research Funding

The most disturbing aspect of the scientific community's perception of declining research project grant support is that it predisposes against significant corrections for other elements of the research base. *The committee concluded that this has led to a climate where federal support for health sciences research has become focused too heavily on projects and not enough on developing career scientists and fostering creative environments.* That is, over the last decade training, equipment, and facilities have become steadily and significantly underfunded in relation to research project support. Unfortunately, funding from other nonfederal sources, although substantial, has not compensated sufficiently for the accumulated loss of federal support for these long-term investments in the health sciences research enterprise. Before recommending the steps that can begin to address these accumulated imbalances, the committee reviews briefly in the next section some of the additional analytic factors that must be considered as propagating the specific status of the neglected health research components—namely, training, equipment, and facilities.

Support for Training

Many of today's senior health science faculty members in colleges, universities, and medical centers can trace their careers to the various training programs underwritten by NIH/ADAMHA between 1950 and 1970. However, federal funds allocated for training new researchers have not kept pace with expanding research opportunities. As indicated in Figure 4-9, NIH support for training as a percent of the extramural budget declined from 17.2 percent in 1970 to 6.6 percent in 1978 and even further to 4.2 percent in 1988. Furthermore, inflationary pressures have been shrinking the real dollar value of stipends awarded to trainees and fellows.

The emergence of unexpected health crises, such as AIDS, emphasizes the importance of maintaining a cadre of highly talented scientific personnel who can be redirected quickly as needed. According to a recently released report by the Office of Science and Engineering Personnel of the National Research Council, *Biomedical and Behavioral Research Scientists: Their Training and Supply,*[1] entrants into health sciences research have increased slightly while recruitment of Ph.D. scientists by the private sector has increased markedly. Furthermore, predictions of an increasing attrition rate among scientists trained during the postwar expansion is cause for concern about research personnel shortages before the end of this century. These and other factors will affect the pool of educators and mentors to train the next generation of scientists, in both academia and industry.

The committee concludes that steps must be taken now to maintain the pool of career scientists by recruiting and retaining the best possible candidates. Resource allocation policies fostering health research careers will require long-term investments from a variety of sources. Academia, government, industry, private foundations, and voluntary health agencies need to play cooperative roles in developing and pursuing effective strategies for enhancing and renewing the nation's health sciences talent base. These strategies should not only focus on recruiting individuals into science careers, but should also nurture these individuals to the level where they become independent young investigators. New approaches should include programs targeted at multidisciplinary and interdisciplinary training of scientists who are becoming increasingly necessary for addressing complex health questions.

The federal government along with the scientific community must acknowledge the need for continued recruitment and take responsibility for developing new talent to ensure the future vitality of the health sciences enterprise. This committee acknowledges that funding for talent development may not be available from new congressional allocations for NIH and ADAMHA. The committee is also deeply concerned that any redistribution of existing funds from research project support will increase pressures on the funding picture. *Nevertheless, the committee believes that the scientific community must show commitment to the long-term integrity of the overall system, even if that means short-term sacrifices to research allocations in order to reinvigorate training and replenish the scientific talent pool.*

Support for Equipment and Facilities

The committee concluded that inadequate or unsuitable space and obsolete equipment have restricted the number and types of research projects that can be undertaken. Although the extent of the needs for construction, repair, and renovation of health sciences research facilities is difficult to determine, estimates run as high as $8 billion. The committee believes the long-term decline in federal programs for research facility construction and equipment renewal is partially responsible for deterioration of the nation's research laboratories. Consequently, the committee believes that these worsening conditions potentially could have adverse affects on research training and the productivity level of the nation's scientific workforce.

Federal support for research facilities has diminished drastically over the past two decades. Federal grant programs in the 1960s were very successful in expanding the nation's research capabilities, but several factors caused the NIH and National Science Foundation (NSF) facilities programs to be eliminated in the early 1970s. For instance, the increasing commitment of resources to the Vietnam War severely strained domestic programs, including facilities programs at academic institutions. Also, OMB (at that time known as the Bureau of the Budget) began pressuring NSF and NIH to justify continuing expansion of the nation's research facilities at a time when both college enrollments and the growth in federal R&D funds were leveling off. This forced a policy of supporting facilities solely through indirect cost recovery associated with research project grants.

Except for some limited appropriations for AIDS research facilities, federal funds for health research facilities have been negligible over the past 10 years. This continued neglect comes at a time of escalating maintenance costs, increasing regulatory standards, increasing technological sophistication, and a dramatic growth in scientific opportunities. Although some state governments and the private sector continue to make significant contributions to support the physical infrastructure for health research, they cannot be expected to meet the total demand. Clearly, there is a need to establish a national policy for renewal and expansion of the health sciences research infrastructure.

The committee concluded that despite repeated studies calling for increased support for research facilities, no long-term federal strategy exists to restore the physical infrastructure for health research. There is no consensus within government or the research community on the need for expanded versus renovated facilities, the best mechanism for program support, or the respective roles of the interested sponsoring parties. Additionally, there is no mechanism to coordinate the various independent contributors supporting facilities and equipment. Without a clear set of goals and a cohesive national policy, U.S. universities and research institutions will continue to decay and will be forced to seek short-term solutions to their facilities' needs by soliciting pork barreled appropriations from Congress.

TOWARD A POSITIVE RESEARCH ENVIRONMENT

The committee believes that the goals of health research can be achieved only by creating a positive research environment for health sciences. This environment should

• identify and encourage young, talented individuals to pursue health research careers;
• provide stable research support for talented scientists throughout their careers;
• offer flexibility in allocating resources to foster creativity and meet changing demands; and
• provide the modern laboratories and equipment necessary for scientific research and training.

These characteristics, in turn, require effective coordination and leadership from the federal research agencies; competent, objective public and private sector administration; and responsiveness to the wishes of the American people through the political process.

When the environment is positive, supportive, and reasonably predictable, it nurtures innovative research. A congenial environment is equally important, for it encourages talented people to seek careers in health research while fostering the careers of established scientists. The continued vitality of health sciences research requires a system of stable support for scientists but with the flexibility to allocate resources in order to meet changing demands. The committee believes that while the scientific community must be held accountable for use of federal research funds, there has to be stable support and flexible policies to promote an optimal research environment.

General Research Funding Guideline

To place the existing research establishment into an economic perspective, the committee analyzed each component in terms of capital investment relative to its productive life expectancy. The committee determined the following: (1) individual scientists are the most vital long-term investment in the research system; (2) capital investment in facilities is of a slightly shorter duration; and (3) individual research projects and the equipment used by researchers generally are the shortest and the most variable investment relative to time.

A certain degree of flexibility is necessary for supporting the components of the research enterprise. This fundamental principle implies that support for one component can be reduced for a brief period of time in order to provide funds to invigorate another component. The committee ascertained that those elements with the longest survival value (namely the research workforce and facilities) may be resilient enough to withstand temporary budget freezes or slight reductions in order to accommodate the immediate needs of components with shorter investment periods (research projects and equipment). Although short-term exigencies that favor support for one component over the others may be necessary for brief periods, continuance of such short-term policies will, in time, undermine the integrity of the entire system. In practice, emphasis on the short term needs of the research enterprise has led to underemphasis of funding for the training pipeline and facilities.

The committee concluded that the guiding principle for maintaining long-term balance within the system is adequate support for each component. At any given level of federal funding, support for each component must be calculated relative to society's expectations of the entire research enterprise.

Recommendation 1: The committee recommends that Congress, NIH and ADAMHA administrators, and scientists employ a priority-setting framework for allocating funds to meet long- and short-term research needs in order to correct and maintain the appropriate overall balance among the individual components of the research establishment (people, projects, and facilities).

To meet the health science research goals at any given level of overall support, relative amounts of support must be designated for the separate but interlocking components of the research system. The overriding objective of maintaining the integrity of a vigorous research system must be considered in all short-term decisions. Short- and long-term research goals must be defined not only by the amount of money allocated to perform specific research projects, but consideration also must be given to the number of researchers that will be necessary in the future, their equipment needs, and the adequacy of the facilities in which the research is to be performed. Thus, if the future requirements for investigators, facilities, and the amount of research can be estimated, the amount of funds necessary for each component to sustain a viable system can be calculated. Once projections of support needs for each component are determined, these estimates can be used to make a judgment as to what proportion of the total research budget should be designated for each component.

Therefore, several interlocking levels of priority setting and decision making must be considered when allocating research funds.

- The total appropriations to all federal agencies receiving funds for health sciences research, including NIH and ADAMHA;
- the allocations within each institute of NIH/ADAMHA for research and training needs; and
- the allocations within specific research program areas (generally, disease areas such as leukemia within the National Cancer Institute [NCI] or acute myocardial infarction within the National Heart, Lung and Blood Institute [NHLBI]).

This can be interpreted to mean that each program division of each institute or agency will have specific programmatic needs to accomplish their mission at any given level of support. With established goals an estimated amount of investigators, research facilities, and research projects (with equipment as a proportion of project funds) will be required over a period of time. The desired balance among the components will differ depending on the area of research being supported. Considering that the research establishment is made up of a series of such long-term goals, it will be necessary to (1) replenish a certain percentage of talented investigators; (2) renovate or replace a certain percentage of buildings or renew equipment; and (3) support a certain level of research activity in order to preserve the integrity of the overall system and attain long-term goals.

The committee did not attempt to focus on the substantive programmatic directions of the individual institutes nor their reasons for selecting, continuing, or redirecting their programmatic emphases. Each institute already has in place both a Board of Scientific Counselors that oversees the intramural program and a congressionally mandated National Advisory

Council that oversees the extramural program. Additionally, there are program advisory boards in many institutes that help define specific program objectives and research directions. In principle, the councils and associated advisory boards are responsible for extramural program planning and setting program priorities.

Criteria for resource allocation at each of these levels should, however, be amenable to application of the principles and guidelines enunciated here. Each decision requires an estimate of the existing knowledge available to achieve the goal, the existing cadres of investigators needed to do so, and the availability of facilities and equipment to carry out these studies. Calculations must take into consideration the current capabilities of the research system (e.g., how much repair is necessary on the existing facilities, or, questions such as are there enough of the needed specialists to conduct the research). Next, projections must be made for annual targets toward achieving the determined goals within an established time period (for example, if 1,000 more investigators trained for a particular research field are needed by the year 2000, outlays for 100 more researchers annually for the next 10 years will be required). Once these objectives and programs have been funded, their implementation then devolves to the final two steps of the allocation process: (1) the allocation of awarded grant funds for a specific research project contributing to the goals of the research program and (2) the total allocation of funds to the specific universities, hospitals and research institutions that will assume fiscal responsibility for the funds, administer them, and provide the infrastructure for the research projects.

The objective of this framework is not to produce one overriding formula that can be applied across the spectrum. Rather, it is to allow for determining priorities among competing needs within different research areas. This framework serves as a guideline for determining particular research needs from the bottom up. The committee emphasizes the importance of designing a process that allows flexibility in order to meet a variety of needs, both among various research programs as well as within specific research areas. **The committee also emphasizes the need for continuous monitoring of talent development within research programs so that this information can be provided to coordinating advisory bodies such as the Federal Coordinating Council for Science, Engineering, and Technology, (FCCSET) and a forum like the Government-University-Industry Research Roundtable (GUIRR) (see recommendations 6.1 and 6.2 below).**

Rebalancing of Health Sciences Research Funds

The committee has concluded that allocation policies over the past two decades have forced an overall imbalance in the health sciences research system in which support for research project grants has been heavily favored at the expense of training and facilities. Reestablishing balance among research, training, and facilities is crucial in order for the United States to maintain a vigorous research enterprise and sustain international preeminence in health research. In order to rebalance the system, the committee employed the preceding framework to analyze the status of long-term capital investment among the components of the research base.

In order to make up for past deficiencies in training allocations throughout the 1980s, and to meet higher personnel demands towards the end of the 1990s, the committee feels that an accelerated growth of the training budget is necessary. The committee emphasizes that there is an integral relationship between research and training. Since an estimated one-quarter of NIH and ADAMHA support for research training is accomplished indirectly through research project grants, allocation policy can not be separated easily into research and training components. However, for defining allocation policy, and in the absence of better data on research project grant funded training, these functions can be treated independently. The committee feels the research community must develop and implement corrective strategies now to avert a workforce crisis later in this decade.

To address the funding imbalances, the committee developed allocation strategies under four budget scenarios for balanced funding through the 1990s: (1) no real growth in the health sciences research budget (i.e., no growth beyond inflation), (2) 2 percent annual real growth, (3) 4 percent annual real growth, and, (4) possible allocation strategies for budgetary growth higher than 4 percent.

Recommendation 2: The committee recommends that federal health research funds be reallocated over the next 10 years according to the suggested percentages in the growth scenarios outlined below.

1. No Real Growth: Even in the event of no average real growth in the health sciences research budget during the 1990s, the committee recommends that funds for training the next generation of health scientists be increased incrementally from 4.20 to 5.75 percent of the total extramural research budget by 1995 and 6.75 percent by the year 2000. Concurrently, the committee recommends that extramural construction funds be increased incrementally from the present 0.25 percent of the extramural budget to 0.50 percent by 1995 and that this level be maintained through the end of the decade.

This redistribution of funds to training and facilities should come from increased congressional appropriations and not reduce the pool of funds for research (Figures 7-1 and 7-2 and Appendix Table A-22). However, in real terms (dollars adjusted for inflation) there will be a slight reduction of research funds under this proposal. The proposal calls for shifting 0.20 percent of the research budget (or about $12 million constant dollars per year) to the training budget each year for the next decade. With an

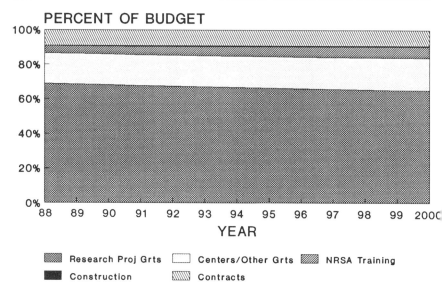

FIGURE 7-1   Percentage reallocation of the NIH extramural budget under both no real growth or two percent real growth scenarios.

average cost per full-time training position (FTTP) equivalent of $24,000, this proposal would reallocate enough funds to increase FTTPs by nearly 400 per year. **The committee believes that this growth in the training budget will not enlarge the research project grant applicant pool; rather, the net effect of this gradual reallocation will be to replace the increasing number of scientists expected to retire later this decade.** Furthermore, this recommendation parallels that recommended in the NRC report *Biomedical and Behavioral Research Scientists: Their Training and Supply.*[1]

The minor shift of funds for extramural construction will merely allow the NIH to meet the most urgent facilities crises. **The committee cannot recommend shifting larger proportions of federal health sciences research funds into the construction category at a time when an increasing number of research grants are not funded fully.** On the other hand, the complete absence of funds authorized for construction could jeopardize the building and renovation of facilities crucial to scientific progress.

The committee recommends that a small percentage of funds be restored to the centers and other grants category over the next decade as well. The proportion of extramural funds committed to centers declined steadily throughout the 1980s, and continued decline in support could diminish the quality of the research conducted in these environments. It becomes all the more important to increase the support for centers that can serve as technology transfer sites for the translation of research results into clinical practice. Funds transferred to this category could be used for the growing

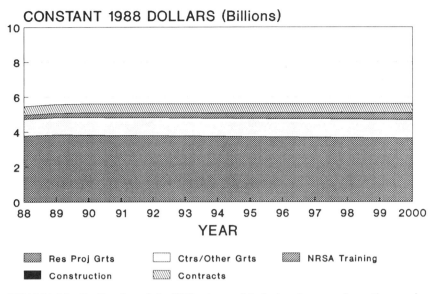

FIGURE 7-2   Reallocation of the NIH extramural budget under no real growth scenario.

number of interdisciplinary and multicenter disease prevention and epidemiological studies. Also included in this budget category under other grants, are the funds for the Biomedical Research Support Grant (BRSG) program. Providing more funds through the BRSG program could enhance the abilities of research institutions to assist their young investigators at the local level and may help stabilize the research efforts of mid-career scientists if the traditional grant system becomes even more unpredictable (see recommendation 4.6).

Shifting funds away from research to training and facilities will have some negative ramifications. Over the next decade, the cost of these reallocations will be about $20 million (constant dollars) per year out of an annual $3.8 billion research project grant budget (1988 total). Since these funds would be reallocated from a variety of research programs, the reductions in the traditional (R01) investigator-initiated research project grant pool would be minimized.

2. Two Percent Real Growth: In the event that the health sciences research budget grows, in real terms, an average of 2-percent annually, the committee again recommends that funds should be reallocated to training and facilities in the same proportions as in the zero growth scenario— training funds increased incrementally from 4.20 to 5.75 percent of the total extramural research budget by 1995 and 6.75 percent by 2000, and extramural construction funds should be increased incrementally from the

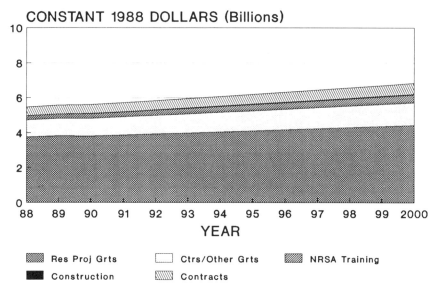

FIGURE 7-3 Reallocation of the NIH extramural budget under a two percent real growth scenario.

present 0.25 percent of the extramural budget to 0.50 percent by 1995 and through the end of the decade. The real growth in the budget in concert with the reallocations will add more funds to training and facilities budgets without decreasing the research grant budget.

Under this scenario, if the NIH budget grows by 2 percent annually in real terms (equivalent to the average annual real growth in the NIH budget throughout the 1980s), the committee feels that portions of the net increase also should be shifted to training and facilities (Figures 7-1 and 7-3 and Appendix Table A-23). Since there has been no real growth in the training budget throughout the 1980s, the committee believes that these recommended percentages of reallocated funds will reestablish NIH's and ADAMHA's leadership in training. The net growth would allow for increasing the number of FTTPs, but the committee feels that some of these augmented training allocations should be used to improve training programs and to address insufficient stipend levels (see recommendation 3 below). The percentage of the research budget allocated to facilities will not change from the zero-growth scenario since proportionately more funds will be available due to growth in the overall budget; and, in any case, the amounts needed to reach the estimated facilities construction requirement (see chapter 6) cannot be drawn from the existing sums.

The committee emphasizes that these reallocations will preserve the same or higher level of research effort by not reducing the research portion of the budget in real terms. In fact, if the average size of research project grants remains constant ($184,000 in 1988) through the next decade, the total number of grants supported by NIH could potentially grow from the present level of 20,300 to nearly 24,000. Although the number of funded research grants will grow by about 360-370 per year over the decade, the success rate for applicants will remain relatively unchanged (presently about 24 percent) if the annual number of applications continues to exceed the present 19,500 level.

3. Four Percent Real Growth: In the event that the health sciences research budget grows an average of 4 percent annually, the committee recommends that funds for training be increased incrementally from 4.20 percent to approximately 5.4 percent of the total extramural research budget by 1995 and to 6.2 percent by 2000. Reallocation of funds for construction should follow the same pattern as the two previous scenarios: an incremental increase of construction funds to 0.50 percent of the extramural budget.

The target percentages for funds to be reallocated to training under the 4 percent growth scenario are somewhat smaller than the figures in the 2 percent and zero growth scenarios (Figures 7-4 and 7-5 and Appendix Table A-24). Although the overall percentage of the extramural budget committed to training is less under this scenario, the funding level actually would increase more rapidly because of the real growth in the overall budget. Obviously, faster growth of the training budget would eventually outpace the resources available to support the net increase in researchers.

A 4 percent annual real growth in research funds would allow for a modest expansion of the research base over the next ten years. The net increase in available research funds would allow for the overall number of NIH research project grants to expand gradually, at a rate of about 1000 per year at 1988 grant sizes from the present 20,300 to about 29,400. In 1991 alone, this would raise the annual number of new and competing awards to approximately 6,000. However, with applications exceeding 19,500 and expected to go even higher, the annual success rate will only approach 28 to 30 percent. The committee believes that even at this pace of budget growth a large number high quality research proposals will go unfunded.

4. More Rapid Growth: The committee also considered the possibility that the NIH budget would grow at a more rapid pace, and what the longer term ramifications of such growth might be. The committee was convinced from the data and testimony it received that if all grant parameters (i.e., average grant size and duration, and the annual number of applications) were to remain constant the national health research effort could effectively utilize resources growing at a much higher rate. A larger research effort could build more effectively and rapidly upon the previous accomplishments

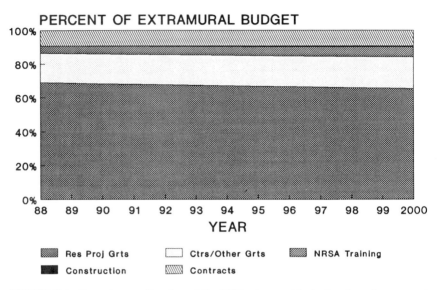

FIGURE 7-4   Percentage reallocation of the NIH extramural budget under a four percent real growth scenario.

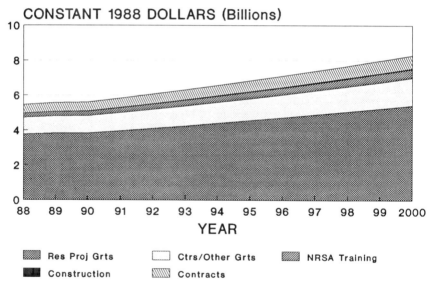

FIGURE 7-5   Reallocation of the NIH extramural budget under a four percent real growth scenario.

in health research and further broaden our knowledge of human biology and disease. For example, simply to regain the 35 percent grant success rate that existed between 1980 and 1987, would require funds for approximately 7,000 new and competing awards annually. Using the allocation proportions described above, would require an 8 per cent annual real growth.

The overall allocation of funds among extramural research projects, training, and facilities will depend upon the particular needs of the scientists performing research within various scientific programs and disciplines, and the granting mechanisms deployed to meet the goals of these research programs. The committee's suggested allocations are directed towards the overall distribution of funds in order to strengthen the research enterprise by ensuring adequate, but balanced support to all components of the research enterprise. The committee has not specifically examined the proportion of funds expended on intramural research within any given NIH/ADAMHA institute. This issue has been examined recently by another IOM study group. Growth in the intramural programs is guided by program objectives and advisory councils' oversight, and is constrained by space limitations and employment ceilings.

Within these guidelines, the committee emphasizes that any funds to be redistributed should be drawn first from increases in the annual federal appropriations. However, even in the event of no real growth in the federal health research budget, the committee firmly endorses that incremental increases in training funds be reallocated from the nominal increases in the overall extramural budget (funds not adjusted for inflation). Under circumstances of real growth, the proposed training increases should come from the new funds so as to detract minimally from the ongoing research effort. Furthermore, the committee emphasizes the importance of making gradual reallocations in order to maintain research support stability.

The committee is aware that this proposal may not be received favorably by the scientific community at a time when research grants are not funded fully and research careers appear to be in jeopardy. Although the committee recognizes that these short-term problems abound, it is making these recommendations for the long-term integrity of the research enterprise. The earlier Institute of Medicine (IOM) report, *Resources for Clinical Investigation*,[2] has recommended that 1,000 clinical investigation training positions be made available. Additionally, the next biomedical and behavioral manpower report by the NRC scheduled to be released in 1992 is expected to review closely the need for increasing the number of physician-scientists as well as the scientific doctoral pool. If the federal research budget grows in real terms and if continued monitoring by the National Research Council (NRC) Committee on Biomedical and Behavioral Workforce Needs demonstrates an increasing demand for physician-scientists, the proposed shift of funds to the training budget would make resources available for implementing these changes. Additionally, adjustments to the research granting system presented below are designed to stabilize research careers through additional steps and to ensure a vigorous, albeit constrained, health research establishment.

TALENT RENEWAL

It has been argued that there are already too many grant applicants not receiving federal funds and that training more will only exacerbate this problem. However, the committee believes that the United States must take a prospective view of the anticipated scientific work force demands for the next 20 to 30 years. There are strong indications that the failure to recruit new people into the health sciences and to compete with other more secure or appealing career lines will significantly hamper the United States' ability to confront future health research challenges. Furthermore, given the likelihood that retirements and other sources of attrition are on the rise, it becomes all the more imperative to address training needs immediately.

Recommendation 3: The committee recommends an approach to restore balance in the development of scientific talent through a broad spectrum of incentives and encouragements. The committee stresses that strategies must be developed to

1. **recruit undergraduate students into the health sciences;**
2. **increase the interest of underrepresented groups, including women and minorities, in careers in health science research;**
3. **enhance the continuum of support mechanisms for graduate students;**
4. **improve the training of physician-scientists; and**
5. **devote additional attention to the needs of younger scientists.**

Increasing the Attraction of Health Science Research Careers for Undergraduates

Recommendation 3.1: The committee recommends that programs be supported by the National Science Foundation (NSF) and other federal agencies, along with the private sector, to introduce undergraduates to career opportunities in health sciences research.

The challenge of preparing and motivating students to pursue health science careers begins at the level of primary education. According to several recent studies, there has been a decline in the mathematics and science competencies of U.S. students from kindergarten through twelfth grade. Although the present study was not intended to address K through 12 education, the committee feels it is important to recognize that the development of future scientists begins in elementary school—not at the time of college enrollment.

Major losses to the science and engineering talent pool occur during the undergraduate years—when career decisions usually are made. Throughout the 1950s and 1960s, the primary source of federal support for undergraduate science education was the Science and Engineering Education (SEE) Directorate of the NSF. In the early 1960s the SEE budget swelled to 46 percent of the entire NSF budget. However, by 1983 only 1.5 percent of the total NSF budget was committed to this directorate. Recent efforts to reemphasize the importance of federal support for science and mathematics education has resulted in the budget for SEE growing from $55 million in 1987 to a proposed $251 million in the 1991 budget—nearly 10 percent of the NSF Budget. Students interested in the health sciences need to be introduced to research opportunities that will encourage them to continue these studies in graduate or medical school. While undergraduate science education falls within the purview of the NSF, the committee believes that research experiences for undergraduates pursuing careers in the health sciences cannot be addressed sufficiently by that agency alone. *The committee concluded that programs sponsored by the federal government, foundations, and voluntary health agencies are necessary to encourage and support students pursuing careers in health research.*

These programs should include research experience in association with faculty members who can serve as role models and mentors. Several programs, including NSF's Research Experience for Undergraduates (REU) and Research at Undergraduate Institutions (RUI) programs, Congress's National Scholars Program, and the Howard Hughes Medical Institute's donations to liberal arts colleges, have been developed and provide frameworks that could be expanded to improve the flow of undergraduates into the health sciences. These types of programs provide incentives for investigators to become more involved in undergraduate research training and mentoring, and they offer stimuli for students to pursue careers in scientific research.

Considerable discussion within the committee focused on establishing programs through NIH and ADAMHA to provide supplemental research grant monies to support the involvement of undergraduate students in research project grants—similar to NSF's REU and RUI programs. Such programs would provide students with research experience while they are making career choices. This should increase the chances that many of the students involved in this type of research will go on to choose health research careers. The committee recognizes the merits of these types of undergraduate science programs, which have traditionally been within the purview of the NSF and the Department of Education. Whereas a few members of the committee felt strongly that NIH and ADAMHA should invest more resources at the undergraduate stage of the pipeline, the majority of the committee concluded that in a no growth budget reallocation of existing funds for undergraduate programs could not be justified. However, in the event of real growth in the federal research budget, various undergraduate health research training models will merit additional attention.

Enhancing the Attractiveness of Health Science Careers for Women and Minorities

Recommendation 3.2: The committee recommends that programs be developed by the federal government and the private sector that are designed to encourage more women and minorities to pursue careers in the health sciences.

Of particular concern with regard to undergraduate science enrollment is the underparticipation of women and minority students. Although these students may be sufficiently prepared for a science and engineering education when they begin their college studies, they choose these avenues of study in significantly lower proportions than similarly prepared white males. Undergraduate programs specifically designed to encourage women and minority students to pursue their scientific career aspirations could reverse this trend and significantly increase their numbers.

Similar to the health sciences research opportunities program described in the above recommendation, a key element to the success of these programs is undergraduate exposure to research under the guidance of faculty members or through collaboration with a graduate program or medical school. Currently, the federal government supports programs to increase participation of minority undergraduates in health sciences through awards to specific institutions. The NIH Minority Access to Research Careers (MARC) program for undergraduate experiences in research provides a model for introducing these students to careers in the health sciences.

The committee believes that the current system neglects the diversity of individual needs of students in these underrepresented groups. The design of successful programs to address this issue should include support that is available to any qualified student, regardless of his or her choice of school. Support should be focused on the abilities of the individual and the research and training programs of the host institution including those institutions serving predominantly minority students. Thus, program expansion should emphasize fellowships and faculty involvement within every college and university. Programs that meet the needs of the individual students should help increase the number of students from underrepresented groups who go on to graduate studies in the health sciences.

Reestablishing Competitive Predoctoral Support

Recommendation 3.3: The committee recommends that NIH and ADAMHA reestablish a competitive predoctoral fellowship program for individuals.

The committee believes that there is an imbalance in NIH and ADAMHA support for graduate studies in the health sciences. The current system heavily favors institutional training grants over individual fellowships. The committee believes, however, that a combination of mechanisms to support predoctoral students throughout their studies is important.

In the 1960s the portion of the NIH training portfolio devoted to predoctoral fellowships accounted for more than 8 percent of the training budget. The National Research Service Act in 1974 almost eliminated this type of training support, shifting the emphasis to predoctoral training grants and away from fellowships awarded to individual students attending institutions of their own selection. Currently, predoctoral fellowships account for less than 2 percent of all NIH training money (about 200 positions out of approximately 11,000 full-time equivalents). One variable in the committee's analysis is the extent of pre- and postdoctoral training support provided through research project grants. One estimate shows that the number of trainees supported on research project grants has nearly doubled between 1979 and 1987—from 2673 to 4426. Without accurate data, which is not collected by the NIH, the committee's recommendations can address only the mix of support within the training and fellowship programs.

Most of the committee agrees that there would be a number of advantages to reinstituting a predoctoral fellowship program. Students would be supported directly, allowing them more freedom to select the area of investigation they wish to pursue. Students would apply for these graduate fellowships in a national competitive process, similar to procedures used for NIH postdoctoral fellowships. Thus, student support would not be connected directly with renewal of investigator research project support. Most importantly, direct fellowship awards to students would provide a strong signal that the student is an integral and valued member of the health sciences research enterprise, which would enable more aggressive recruitment of students into postbaccalaureate education and training in the health sciences. The committee emphasizes that the underparticipation of minorities and women also must be addressed within this program as well.

Improving the Training of Physicians for Research Careers

Recommendation 3.4: The committee recommends that the number of physician investigators—active and in training—be assessed. Assuming a real decline in the number of physician-scientists, the committee further recommends reallocating resources in order to create a more formal system for training physician-scientists, including curriculum requirements. In addition, experimental federally funded training programs in clinical research and public health research also should be established.

The committee is concerned about the apparent inability to recruit sufficient numbers of physicians into scientific careers, especially clinical investigator careers. The physician-scientist is the critical link between the knowledge uncovered in the laboratory and the translation of that knowledge into clinical practice. However, various indicators, such as the proportion of NIH grants awarded to physician investigators and the numbers of physicians reporting research activities, have shown a steady decline in physician-scientist numbers since the early 1970s.

The committee believes it is essential to have physician-scientists engaged in both basic and clinical research. Recruiting physicians into research careers is hampered severely by the length of time necessary for clinical training as well as the difficulty of conducting research during this training period. Additionally, the current unfocused structure of many physician research training experiences does not introduce trainees sufficiently to scientific project design, research methodology, and statistical analysis.

Particularly troublesome is the apparent decline in the number of physicians pursuing clinical research. A recent IOM study committee closely examined the resources available for clinical investigation and the complex issues involved in attracting physicians into clinical research. The study group concluded that the data were inadequate regarding the nature of clinical research and level of support in this country. However, the study group was able to identify several barriers to individuals pursuing careers in clinical investigation.

The committee believes there is a "triple threat" to academic physicians in the posttraining years: they are expected to be exceptional researchers, exceptional clinicians, and exceptional teachers and mentors. These pressures probably have discouraged many physicians from remaining actively engaged in research and will have to be alleviated in order to interest more physicians in research careers.

The committee believes that formal training for physician-scientists should include experience in scientific research protocol design, research

methodology, epidemiology, and statistical analysis. A 1- or 2-year research experience, particularly when poorly focused, often leaves physician-
scientists less competitive than Ph.D. scientists on peer-reviewed grant applications. Therefore, a national program for training physician-scientists
should encourage more physicians to pursue research careers, and improve
their success in the competitive grant system.

The committee supports the recommendation of the recent IOM report *Resources for Clinical Investigation* that federal funds be allocated for
creating a national program for training clinical researchers. In addition,
the committee believes this should include the aforementioned curriculum
requirements and require matching funds from medical schools. This program should be assessed and analyzed periodically for its effectiveness in
recruiting and retaining more M.D. scientists in clinical investigation.

Possibly another way to enhance the training of physician-scientists
is by expanding NIH's Medical Scientist Training Program (MSTP). This
program facilitates obtaining both an M.D. and a Ph.D. degree in a health-
related science. **To encourage adequate training of physician-scientists, the
committee encourages NIH to expand the MSTP program. The committee
also supports ADAMHA in its efforts to initiate a similar program.** The
committee believes that the MSTP program provides valuable training
experiences for physician-scientist trainees at a crucial period in their
scientific career development. In addition, M.D./Ph.D. training support
should be available through individual grants as well as through institutional
training grants, analogous to doctoral training programs.

Improving the Opportunities for Young Investigators

**Recommendation 3.5: The committee recommends that NIH and
ADAMHA modify their FIRST award programs to incorporate a formalized
assessment of progress by a scientific panel in the third year.**

Once talented individuals have spent many years successfully training
for a research career, they should have confidence they will be able to
gain entry into the research system. Frequent proposal writing to obtain
small project grants can prevent young investigators from developing a
solid, long-term line of investigation. Also, the committee believes that the
transitional period between postdoctoral training and established scientist
is the most crucial in getting young, creative minds into productive research
careers.

As competition in the traditional research project grant system increased through the late 1970s and early 1980s, many in the scientific
community felt that grant applications from young investigators were at a
competitive disadvantage in peer review. Since many of these individuals
had not established their own lines of investigation and were inexperienced

at writing concise and lucid grant applications, their applications may not have been received as favorably as those from senior scientists.

To provide these young applicants access to the federal research grant system, NIH, and later ADAMHA, initiated a program aimed specifically at the posttrainee/prescientist career stage called the First Independent Research Support and Transition (FIRST) award. The FIRST award program guarantees awardees 5 years of support and a maximum of $350,000. These longer award periods for young investigators provide stability and the additional time often needed to set up new laboratories. However, no funds are set aside regularly for these awards, which means there is no assurance that FIRST grant applications will be awarded when the researcher is ready to apply for one. In effect, these young investigators continue to compete head on in peer review with other types of grant applications, namely traditional R01 investigator-initiated grant applications.

The committee feels strongly that these awards are moving in the right programmatic direction for providing entry into the competitive traditional grant system (R01) for young scientists. However, modifications of the FIRST program may be warranted in order to provide more guidance throughout the award period as well as to establish greater similarities to the R01 grant program.

Considering the nature of the FIRST award, the committee does not feel that the progress of these awardees should or could be comparable to that required in the traditional R01 system. This rereview should *not* be construed as a contingency for further funding. Rather, it should ensure that FIRST investigators are being indoctrinated properly into independent scientific investigation and prepared to compete for R01s. Furthermore, this should provide an opportunity to redirect the young investigator (if necessary) and ensure that the product of this research will, in fact, enhance the body of medical knowledge. A similar funding mechanism comparable to the FIRST award could be envisioned for midcareer scientists seeking additional training in a new field.

IMPROVING THE RESEARCH PROJECT GRANTS SYSTEM

To carry out this program of talent renewal without compromising the research base, the research project system needs, in the committee's view, some adjustments in order to preserve the existing pool of talented scientists as well. Policies that affect research project support should provide flexibility for responding rapidly to changing research needs but also should provide stable support for productive research scientists.

Modifying Research Project Grants

As the U.S. health research enterprise has matured, there has been increasingly more competition among the investigators applying for grant funding. The expanding realm of research opportunities, along with the increasingly sophisticated nature of research, has outstripped the effectiveness of the existing peer review process for determining priorities among the cluster of excellent grant applications. Whereas the original design of the peer review system operated well prior to the mushrooming of research opportunities in the 1970s, it is no longer reasonable to believe that minor differences in priority scores are accurate measures for all or nothing funding.

These inconsistencies have been highlighted by the differences in the spread of priority scores among NIH study sections. Consequently, NIH has attempted to address these variations by establishing pay lines according to percentile rankings as opposed to priority scores. Nevertheless, even with these modifications, the funding process still can deny funding for novel or otherwise excellent research applications that happen to fall just below the percentile funding point. The committee feels that these harsh cut-off points are allowing excellent research ideas to go unfunded and that they are potentially demoralizing established researchers whose applications may fall right at the margin for funding.

Even after a research grant has been awarded, the amount of the final funding is subject to a completely arbitrary reduction in the process of downward negotiation, as described previously. This is the system NIH and ADAMHA have adopted to reconcile the funding of research grants to the amount of money received in annual appropriations. As the continuing obligations for NIH and ADAMHA increased by the series of policy changes during the 1980s, the percentage of downward negotiation ballooned from 1 to 2 percent to nearly 12 percent in many NIH/ADAMHA institutes.

Step-Down or Rollover Funding

Recommendation 4.1: The committee recommends that NIH and ADAMHA, as well as other sponsors of research, develop pilot programs to evaluate step-down or rollover funding for selected grant awards.

When a renewal application for an NIH or ADAMHA grant falls just below the cut-off point for funding, a mechanism should be available to allow these meritorious projects to continue for an additional year, possibly with a reduced budget. This would permit resubmitting a clarified proposal while not dismantling the laboratory and losing key personnel. Such a rollover mechanism need not be implemented automatically, and the peer review system could decide on whether research programs were no longer productive and should be stopped.

NIH had "phase-out" procedures in the past that allowed investigators to receive funding during an interim year while an amended competing renewal was being rereviewed. Reestablishing transitional-year awards would reduce the threat that research teams and laboratories will be dismantled completely if support temporarily lapses because of an unsuccessful competitive renewal. A pilot program could evaluate the utility and risks of a transitional funding period during grant renewal. Two possibilities for implementing this concept are

1. Rollover funding: This first transitional scenario would apply to research project grants awarded for periods of 5 or more years. An NIH/ADAMHA review of competing renewal applications would be convened two years before grant termination (e.g., in year 4 of a 5-year grant) and would lead to one of two possible outcomes:

• An accepted application would allow the research project to continue for an additional 5 years. Thus, the renewal award would provide funding for the fifth year plus an additional 4 years, extending the project to 9 years.

• An unsuccessful competing renewal in year 4 would require that the investigator submit an amended competing renewal application in year 5. If the amended application is approved, funding would be continued for years 6 through 10.

2. Step-down funding: Another possible mechanism would be to extend funding for an additional year for those renewal applications that fail to merit adequately high percentile rankings and for which revised renewal applications would be invited by the review committee. In such cases the extension year would be funded at a fixed level, such as 60 percent of the last fully funded award period. This type of program would allow investigators to retain key research staff while a revised grant application was being considered.

These are examples of mechanisms that would allow investigators to participate in two consecutive review cycles prior to losing funding.

A Sliding Scale of Support for Approved Awards

Recommendation 4.2: The committee recommends that NIH and ADAMHA consider modifying the traditional investigator-initiated grant system (R01) to fund grants on a sliding scale based on percentile ranking.

The compression of grant applications receiving high- priority scores and the necessity of determining a single pay line for funding does not necessarily take into consideration the benefits that could be derived from those grant applications at the margins. Furthermore, the committee heard concerns that novel research applications may fall frequently at the margins of the pay line, potentially denying breakthroughs in the medical sciences. The committee believes that the scientific community has to cast a wider net in order to capitalize on excellent opportunities that may fall below the funding cut-off point. In an environment of extreme fiscal constraint and across-the-board downward negotiation, expanding the research base seems unlikely.

A sliding-scale funding mechanism could reinforce and protect the best research projects and reduce the pain inflicted throughout the system from downward negotiation. It also would increase the opportunity to sponsor high quality research proposals that are increasingly falling just below an arbitrarily established pay line. *In effect, the administrative cut would be presented to the scientist at the time the grant is awarded—not episodically and unpredictably throughout the award period.* One suggested plan would scale down the award duration or funding level based on some criteria such as the *percentile* ranking. For example,

- those applications in the top decile would receive full funding,
- those applications in the second decile would receive 90 percent funding,
- those application in the third decile would receive 80 percent funding, and
- those applications in the fourth decile would receive 70 percent funding.

A proposal such as this would not be warranted in an environment where 50 percent of grant applications were funded. However, with award rates at or below 25 percent in most institutes, the committee believes that few options exist to expand the research base. For illustrative purposes, if the R01 research budget were $2.0 billion and the average grant size and length was $175,000 for four years, the total number of R01 grants that could be supported in any one year would be 11,428. The turnover per year would be 2,857 assuming 100 percent funding. If funding were 90 percent, which is in line with the current downward negotiations, the total would grow to 12,698 with an average of 3,175 turning over each year or a gain in projects receiving support of slightly more than 300 per year. By using the proposed sliding scale in this example, about $100 million would be available for funding about 3,850 grants per year or an expansion to about 15,360 total.

For scientists, the security of knowing how much funding actually will be received is far superior to a progressive downward negotiation that slowly compromises all research endeavors and complicates administrative planning by research institutions. This proposal would encourage investigators to set priorities in their own programs according to their funding level, since those with lower percentages of funding would have to choose which aspects of their research to pursue. This would preserve scientific talent by not forcing investigators out of the system in the case of a fund/no fund decision. Furthermore, this strategy might also increase the opportunity for young investigators with novel ideas to gain initial access to the grant system despite inexperience in grant writing.

A Dedicated Mechanism Specifically for Novel Research Proposals

Recommendation 4.3: The committee recommends that NIH and ADAMHA consider revamping the Small Grants program (R03) for funding innovative, high-risk ideas.

The committee is concerned that the peer review system may not effectively identify novel ideas that have the potential for making significant breakthroughs in medical knowledge. Because the system is geared toward building on the accepted body of current knowledge, grant proposals that seek to explore tangential or contradictory theories may not fare well in the priority rankings. As funds have become more constrained, the committee believes that study sections and institutes have become even more disinclined to fund high-risk research proposals.

The committee suggests that NIH and ADAMHA adopt the model of NSF's pilot program called Expedited Awards for Novel Research. This program, begun in the engineering directorate in 1986, was expanded in 1989 to include modified peer review. Awards of up to $50,000 are available to principal investigators with especially innovative ideas. The committee emphasizes that this system should not be viewed as an alternative to the peer review system. Rather, it should be used as an opportunity to support exciting but high-risk research that would otherwise go unfunded.

Changes in Research Management

NIH Director's and ADAMHA Administrator's Emergency Funds

Recommendation 4.4: The committee endorses the recommendation by the IOM group studying the NIH Intramural Research Program that Congress annually appropriate to the director of NIH a discretionary fund of no less than $25 million. A discretionary fund also should be appropriated for the ADAMHA administrator. (The committee acknowledges that the proposal for an NIH director's fund has been submitted in the President's 1991 budget.)

The committee concluded that the dynamic nature of the health research environment frequently requires that monies be available to address emerging problems and/or research needs. The committee found that the directors of the various institutes at NIH and ADAMHA are in a unique position to determine specific areas that require urgent attention and that cannot necessarily wait until the next congressional appropriations cycle. This policy change would strengthen the leadership of NIH and ADAMHA by allowing the directors to address emerging issues and special interinstitute research opportunities. This approach also would improve flexibility and provide the directors with the resources to initiate intramural activities across institute lines, without intruding on the independence of the individual institutes. This proposal has surfaced many times in recent years but has never been approved by OMB. However, the President's budget for fiscal year 1991 includes a $20 million fund for the NIH director. There also is a provision to allow the director to reprogram up to 1 percent of the NIH budget without congressional approval.

Multiple Grant Awards and Grant Size

The committee had lengthy discussions about principal investigators having multiple grant awards. The committee felt that, in many instances, investigators may need more than one grant for their research programs, but the committee also was concerned that large blocks of grant funds could be controlled by a few elite scientists, essentially closing the door on young scientists trying to get into the grant system. However, after considerable discussion, the majority of the committee concluded that the system should not impose arbitrary limits on the number of grants per investigator for fear of denying potentially exciting research. Likewise, artificial ceilings on the size of grants may adversely affect the quality of research by requiring large research projects to be broken down into subparts.

Regulation of either or both of these issues has the potential to stifle creativity and inhibit scientific advancement. However, in an era haunted by concerns for domestic spending constraint, it is incumbent on individual scientists and the peer review system to support the best workers to perform the best science in the most productive environment. Implicit in these evaluations are the amounts of significant effort an investigator has available to devote to the needs of a given project and the staffing required. Clearly, if the scientific community appears to be taking unfair advantage of these loosely regulated areas, congressional or administrative controls are inevitable, as evidenced by the recently implemented salary cap on NIH/ADAMHA sponsored investigators.

Federal Demonstration Project

Recommendation 4.5: The committee recommends that the Federal Demonstration Project be expanded as additional experience becomes available.

The Florida Demonstration Project (FDP) was intended to reduce the administrative burden on grantees by streamlining procedures and reducing costs in the sponsored project system. The primary objectives of the project were to

• standardize postaward administration of federal research grants among the federal agencies to the extent possible;
• eliminate most federal prior approvals for budget reallocation;
• simplify research project management procedures; and
• allow an investigator's collective research program to be treated as one administrative and accounting unit rather than each project as a separate unit.

Initial reactions to the Florida Demonstration Project have been generally quite favorable. As of October 1988, the project was redesignated as the Federal Demonstration Project and was expanded to include 26 institutions. This creative approach is likely to continue to be extremely valuable by allowing scientists to concentrate more on their research than on administrative details.

Research Institutions

Research institutions have always shared the support of health sciences researchers with the federal government and other research sponsors. The recommendations of Vannevar Bush emphasizing federally funded research within academic settings was based, in part, on the preexistence of academic laboratories, research career paths, and the close linkage of research and training. *As federally sponsored research programs have expanded, the committee believes some institutions have exploited federal resources as a means to enlarge their faculties by creating positions that rely entirely upon "soft" funding through research project grants.*

Many research institutions have been resourceful in finding additional institutional monies or philanthropic support for investigator salaries or research support. Despite these efforts, the committee ascertained that many universities and research institutes have been unable to secure adequate flexible resources in order to create stability for their faculties. This situation increases the pressure on scientists to obtain federal support as a foundation for a career in research.

With the growth of health sciences research funds slowing, the committee believes that universities and research institutes should strive to strengthen their commitments to career scientists. To recruit, retain, and augment their research faculties, academic research institutions may need to allocate more internal "hard" funds for the career development needs of young research faculty as well as for those scientists in midcareer. In addition, funds also need to be made available for retraining of older investigators and to offset temporary lapses in external research grant support for established scientists. The committee recognizes that research institutions and universities may find it very difficult to decide how to trade off faculty development for health scientists against other competing institutional needs. However, the committee also believes that a clarification of the institution's objectives would be constructive for the future vitality of these organizations and the realistic appraisals by their faculty of their future opportunities.

Biomedical Research Support Grant

Recommendation 4.6: The committee recommends that NIH continue to fund the BRSG program to universities and research institutions in order to continue flexible program development under institutional control. Furthermore, the committee suggests that the universities and research institutions disburse BRSG funds through faculty peer review groups to support new research initiatives, especially those of young investigators.

The ability of universities and research institutions to reward young talent and preserve ongoing projects increases the sense of career security among researchers. The committee believes that the Biomedical Research Support Grant (BRSG) provides flexibility to university faculty and administrators to support new and ongoing initiatives within their own institutions. The size of these awards is related directly to the amount of project funds received from NIH. These funds are disbursed through various mechanisms at the institutional level. In many cases faculty peer review groups decide the utilization of these funds. The committee believes that the BRSG program has played a significant role in funding young scientists and other institutional initiatives crucial to their overall research and training programs.

The committee recommends that funding for the BRSG program should be maintained to allow universities to make decisions regarding their own faculty research needs and that creation of other block grants for developing and preserving scientific talent should be examined as well. However, funding for BRSG and similar grant programs at NIH and ADAMHA has been a continual target in budget cuts. Early in the 1980s the BRSG program was slated for total elimination by OMB. Between fiscal years 1989 and 1990, the BRSG program suffered a cut of $11 million, falling from $55.2 to $44.4 million, and the proposed 1991 budget intends to reduce this program further to $17 million. The committee feels that this small commitment to flexibility and researcher security is crucial for promoting stability in the careers of health scientists.

RESTORING THE PHYSICAL INFRASTRUCTURE

Increasing regulatory standards are putting added stresses on the ability of institutions to improve facilities and upgrade equipment. Sophisticated equipment for protecting the health of laboratory workers using deadly pathogens and hazardous chemicals sometimes requires large budgetary outlays. As federal regulations for animal care and facilities requirements increase, research institutions must invest heavily to comply. Estimates of the average costs to meet new federal animal regulations run as high as $40,000 per grant.

Inadequate facilities and equipment will have to be corrected gradually, for commitment of a substantial portion of existing federal funding to facilities at this time would create another imbalance in the support mechanism for people and projects. The most direct approach to the infrastructure crisis is increased federal funding for health sciences research facilities and equipment. Many believe that renewed federal support for construction and renovation is necessary and that such a program would help stem the flow of direct appeals by individual institutions to Congress for pork barrel appropriations for specific facility development. Many creative solutions will be required to fill the enormous need to modernize the physical research infrastructure.

Direct Grant Program

Recommendation 5.1: The committee recommends that Congress authorize and appropriate funds for a competitive matching fund construction program to renovate or construct health sciences research facilities, bearing in mind the increased costs of updating facilities to meet recently enacted regulations.

Federal construction programs should focus on renovating existing space as well as funding new construction. Initially, a program could be established without additional appropriations by creating a scientific construction authority and appropriating a portion of the nearly $300 million funnelled by Congress to certain institutions through ad hoc pork barrel amendments. These monies would be subject to a comprehensive merit review, taking into consideration both scientific criteria and appropriate socioeconomic and political criteria. The committee feels strongly that pork barreling does not serve the best interests of the nation in the long run and thus should be avoided.

It is unlikely that any new program will be funded at the same level as the Health Facilities Construction Authority was during the 1960s. The proposed program should allocate matching funds to act as an inducement for attracting private and corporate monies as well as state appropriations.

After reviewing past policy, the committee felt that the federal contribution could be highly leveraged by requiring matching from private and state sources on the order of 1:4 (federal:other). Matching could be done on a sliding scale based on the economic need of the institution as determined by a comprehensive merit review, but it should not exceed a 1:1 ratio. Facility needs do not necessarily conform to the categorical divisions of the individual institutes at NIH or ADAMHA. With limited resources available, coordination of the federal biomedical facility renewal efforts can be accomplished only by the directors of NIH and ADAMHA. Comprehensive review should include input from the institute directors, the White House Office of Science and Technology Policy, Congress, and the scientific community. Such a process should prevent unfair political competition for resources and stem appeals for pork barrel funds.

Indirect Cost Adjustments

Recommendation 5.2: To allow greater flexibility for institutions to address their own facilities needs, the committee recommends that the sponsors of health research modify indirect cost (IDC) calculations in the following ways:

1. The federal government should change federal grant accounting procedures to allow negotiation of separate line items in the IDC recovery rate for facilities renovation and construction separate from that of administrative and library costs.

2. The federal government should increase IDC use allowance to reduce amortization periods for buildings and equipment.

3. Private foundations, voluntary health organizations, and corporations should observe more closely the true costs of the research they sponsor, including the IDC portion.

There are also indirect means by which the federal government and other sponsors of health research can renew the health research infrastructure. Within the federal system the IDC recovery rates for health research conducted at universities and research institutions are negotiated on an individual basis with federal agencies. The allowable depreciation costs for facilities and equipment do not accurately reflect replacement costs. The current version of OMB Circulars A-21 and A-110 allow for building amortization over 50 years (or 2 percent per year) and equipment amortization for 15 years or 6.67 percent per year. From the data available, the committee concluded that this portion of IDC recovery allowances is unrealistic and inadequate.

Another facet of this complex problem is the underpayment of indirect costs by foundations and corporations. By placing caps on the amounts of indirect costs allowable on sponsored research, these sponsors compound IDC recovery problems for colleges and universities. As a result, institutional funds are consumed to support the indirect costs associated with these projects. This constraint may force some institutions to refuse support from these sources if the indirect costs cannot be recouped in a fair and equitable manner.

Many nonprofit sponsors are very concerned about the high IDC rates at the top private research institutions. Paying these high IDC rates easily could consume much of these sponsors' resources available for the direct costs of performing research. However, if universities are forced to transfer indirect costs into direct cost categories, the required funding will remain the same.

Most research buildings become obsolete for conducting sophisticated research in 20 years, and equipment is often obsolete between 4 to 7 years after purchase. The committee feels that sponsors of health research should link support for particular facilities with individual research projects to allow faster recovery of institutional funds used to maintain facilities and to repay loans used for construction or renovation. In order to accomplish this, research institutions need to have options available to recoup previous expenditures for renewing their research physical plant. This could be done by changing the annual IDC allowance for building amortization from the present 2 percent to 5 percent and by raising the allowance for equipment amortization from 6.67 to 20 percent. This would allow research institutions to depreciate their buildings over 20 years rather than 50 and to depreciate equipment in 5 years rather than 15.

The committee emphasizes that this policy change must not reduce the pool of funds available for direct costs and strongly urges universities and other research organizations to keep down the administrative portions of overhead. This seems impossible in light of the increasing federal bureaucratic regulations, but failing to keep these costs in check will inevitably lead to IDC caps and subsequent loss of institutional control over these finances. However, this policy change could allow research institutions more flexibility in setting their own priorities within their budgets for IDC recovery. **The committee also emphasizes that some assurances must be made on the part of the grantee institutions that these funds be sequestered and utilized only for facilities and equipment renewal and not for administrative overhead.** Inaction now will only exacerbate the growing infrastructure problems at colleges and universities.

Creative Financing

Recommendation 5.3: The committee recommends that rules be adjusted so that indirect costs can be applied to direct rental costs of leased facilities.

Alternatives to the traditional forms of capital formation are beginning to reshape the way academia raises money for capital improvements. State and local governments are investing in academic facilities for education and garnering possible economic advantages by providing a sound scientific base in their locales. Partnerships with industry (although limited) are providing an alternative method for capital formation. Patenting and licensing intellectual property also are bringing financial returns that can be invested in facilities at some institutions as well.

The committee heard suggestions that institutions should attempt to offset some of the high costs of research facilities and equipment by entering into cooperative agreements to share resources. Some research institutions recently have developed innovative approaches to develop research facilities by creating long-term arrangements with private developers. By combining off campus IDC rates with direct rental payments, research institutions can enter into such lease arrangements. It is conceivable that in such cases rental payment may provide a means of eventually purchasing the property by the research institution.

In some cases research institutions may wish to lease land to a developer who will construct a research facility. The developer may, in turn, lease the space in the research building back to the research institution. In such cases maximum flexibility should be provided so that the building can be leased or purchased through direct or indirect costs associated with research conducted in the facility. Developer interest in these types of projects may be predicated upon tax accounting rules, which may require some accommodation with regard to how rental or overhead funding is provided.

ESTABLISHING AN ONGOING PROCESS FOR RESEARCH PROGRAM MANAGEMENT AND OVERSIGHT

Federal priorities for health sciences research are determined by the federal budget process through a complex system of interactions among the Executive Branch, Congress, the scientific community, industry, the public, and special interest groups. Ultimately, the federal agenda is set by the funds allocated by Congress through its authorizing, budgeting, and appropriating mechanisms and the recommendations made by Congress in report language. *The committee concluded that the present system is becoming increasingly stressed by short-term corrective actions whose long-term consequences have not been fully assessed.*

Growing federal deficits, earmarking of funds to meet specific health needs, and rigid allocation policies within the health sciences establishment have reduced flexibility within the system. These problems emphasize the need to review federal priorities and to coordinate federal health sciences research efforts. Integration of scientific priorities, as determined by peer review or other review mechanisms, with sound policy will lead to more effective resource allocation, thus improving the overall environment of health sciences research. *Although the committee endorses an open forum for discussing priorities and manners of addressing the problems facing health research, it also emphasizes that top-down research directives will be counterproductive to research.*

Priorities in the private sector are determined in equally complex processes. Whereas many of the larger foundations and voluntary health agencies have boards, steering committees, or a standardized peer review mechanism, others may not have a coordinated means of making decisions according to scientific or other objective criteria. Likewise, corporate R&D decisions are based upon financial determinants in accordance with directives from the boards of directors and stockholders. The committee does not believe that corporate sponsors should be forced to subject their decision making to open peer review, nor would it be possible. However, foundations and corporations should be able to consult with federal policymakers in order to arrive at sound decisions that may complement the federal effort and meet their own needs as well.

Failure to maintain constructive policies that integrate the efforts of government and private and nonprofit sponsors of research will limit scientific progress, jeopardize our continued leadership, and imperil our economic strength. **It is imperative that review and oversight of the balance among the research components be conducted on an ongoing basis.** Therefore, the committee focused on developing mechanisms whereby the sponsors of health sciences research could work cooperatively to monitor progress, develop solutions, and make recommendations to address the problems facing health research highlighted in this report. The objectives of this process are (1) to optimize the use of resources from all sponsors of health sciences research; (2) to improve the nation's capacity to respond to health crises and capitalize on new research opportunities; and (3) to restore balance in the components of the system and resource allocation between support for people, projects, and facilities.

Improving Communication Among the Federal Agencies

Recommendation 6.1: The committee recommends that a Federal

Coordinating Council for Science, Engineering, and Technology (FCCSET) subcommittee for Health Sciences be established to review federal priorities and coordinate federal health sciences research efforts on a continuing basis.

Because of the impact that health-related decisions have on the American public, the committee believes it is essential to continue having high-level health sciences research advice available to the President through the Office of Science and Technology Policy (OSTP). The committee believes that effective mechanisms are necessary for developing cross-cutting health science policy among the federal scientific agencies. As such, the FCCSET provides an excellent model for interagency coordination. FCCSET is composed of the science and technology advisor to the President and one representative from each of the 13 federal agencies sponsoring research. The FCCSET can establish various committees composed of appropriate high-level federal agency representatives to provide a direct link among government agencies, and it can coordinate federal activities.

While the committee believes that the FCCSET will address interagency coordination of research, the White House also needs a formal mechanism for obtaining broad scientific advice from nongovernmental scientists. The current director of OSTP has established a President's Council of Advisors on Science and Technology (PCAST), composed of nongovernmental science experts. *This is the kind of advisory body the committee had in mind, and it is pleased to note the establishment of PCAST as a means of providing the President and FCCSET with advice from nonfederal scientists.*

The health sciences FCCSET committee should use the framework for assessing science and technology budgets proposed in a recent Academy report to evaluate support for health sciences research across federal agencies. The committee should develop guidelines for federal research priorities by considering the following categories from the National Academy of Sciences report *Federal Science and Technology Budget Priorities: New Perspectives and Procedures*[3] as they apply to the health sciences:

- research related to the sponsoring agency's mission;
- health research activities of individual agencies that contribute to the overall science and technology enterprise (including the components of training, fundamental research, and infrastructure);
- cross-cutting research activities of several agencies that contribute to broad national objectives given priority by the President and/or Congress; and
- activities that constitute significant health research initiatives by virtue of their considerable cost.

The committee was pleased to note the appointment of a health scientist last year as the associate director for life sciences within the OSTP and recommends that this associate director be chairman of the proposed FCCSET for Health Sciences. **The committee also recommends that this post continue to be held by individuals with experience in health research and research administration.**

Under the chairmanship of the associate director for life sciences, a special FCCSET committee for health sciences research would bring together the NIH director; ADAMHA administrator; NSF director, health research directors in the Departments of Veterans Affairs, Defense, and Energy; and the heads of the other government agencies sponsoring federal health sciences research programs. These federal agencies would use the guidelines provided by FCCSET to set agency priorities as they pertain to their individual missions. Subsequently, these priorities would be used for budget development by the agencies. The science advisor, in cooperation with the President and director of OMB, then would match program priorities with budget requests to meet the nation's health science research needs.

The committee believes that advice obtained through this mechanism will improve intergovernmental coordination for defining national health sciences research priorities. Ultimately, this will lead to more effective policies for allocating resources for project support, training, equipment, and facilities.

Improving Communication Between Federal and Nonfederal Health Sciences Research Sponsors

Recommendation 6.2: The committee recommends that a forum such as the Government-University-Industry Research Roundtable (GUIRR) be established to review the support of health sciences research on a regular basis and to facilitate communication among the various sectors that support health sciences research.

The vitality of the health sciences research enterprise depends not only upon federal government activities but the cooperation of all parties involved in health sciences research: universities and independent research institutes, as well as the private sector (foundations, voluntary health organizations, and corporations). Each must recognize the interdependence of the various sponsors of health science research in order to maximize its own contributions. These various participants should have a mechanism for open dialogue to facilitate the efficient use of the limited health science research resources.

The GUIRR provides a model for developing a forum to address these issues. The GUIRR was established by the National Academy of Sciences, National Academy of Engineering, and the IOM to address cross-cutting issues that affect all areas of science and technology. It is composed of scientists, engineers, administrators, and policymakers from all sectors with the objectives to understand issues, to inject imaginative thought into the system, and to provide a setting for discussion and the seeking of common ground.

To ensure that the balance of support among components of health sciences research is reestablished and maintained, this review would include evaluation of the relationships among support for research projects, the number of researchers being trained compared to the nation's needs and scientific opportunities, and the status of research facilities. This proposed committee should include representation from the executive and legislative branches of the federal government, pharmaceutical and biotechnology industries, state governments, academic research institutions, private foundations, and voluntary health agencies.

The committee recommends that such a forum initially identify the special responsibilities, interests, and contributions of each of these support sources and explore means to achieve health sciences research goals through greater interaction. The committee also suggests that this group consider sponsoring meetings and workshops or holding public hearings on issues such as

- the special roles and responsibilities of government, industry, and nonprofit organizations in supporting health sciences research;
- the necessity of devising long-term plans to meet next century's research training needs;
- ways to finance the escalating costs for facilities and equipment;
- the appropriate balance of support for research projects, training, and facilities;
- the impact of reallocating resources on the various components of the research enterprise;
- cooperatives among research institutions and the private sector, including review of successes and failures in order to improve new initiatives;
- ways to foster communication among scientists, health practitioners, and corporations to increase technology transfer; and
- long-range planning for health sciences research including formulating a framework to assist establishing 5-, 10- and 20-year goals for individual participants.

After careful consideration of issues that affect all supporters of health sciences research, the proposed GUIRR-like forum should be able to provide information and advice about the needs and activities of the scientific community and their supporters to the proposed FCCSET committee outlined above. This advice would be particularly useful in formulating federal guidelines that include consideration of the need to balance commitments to support investigators directly, to restore facilities and equipment, and to provide training opportunities.

Unresolved Issues to Be Addressed by These Forums

The committee heard a number of complaints about the disease orientation and traditional disciplinary emphasis of federal support for health sciences research, with too little money available for newer fields such as nutrition and prevention research as well as for interdisciplinary projects that do not fit easily into current health research categories. In contrast, the committee also heard strong support for the current system, with the belief that some of these other areas could be handled easily within the existing organizational structure. *However, the charge to this committee did not include an evaluation of the allocation of resources between or among the many topics within the disciplines of health sciences research.*

In a time of intense competition for available resources, where the potential for a national health crisis exists at any time, choices must be made where some fields of research receive more support at the expense of others. Vigorous advocacy by particular special interest groups has had enormous benefit in our democratic decision-making system. However, conflicting views by these groups can confuse decision makers in both the administration and Congress. Such conflicts have made priority setting among competing scientific initiatives extremely difficult. The committee recognizes that it would be advantageous to employ formal and explicit criteria in setting national health priorities and allocating scarce federal resources. Both government science administrators and nonfederal scientific advisory groups could benefit in their decision-making considerations from such criteria.

The science advisors in the White House OSTP, along with the proposed health FCCSET, should work closely with PCAST, NIH/ADAMHA administrators and advisory groups, and the proposed GUIRR-like committee to determine appropriate criteria for setting priorities among fields within the health sciences disciplines and for evaluating new initiatives. This would not be a means to rate competing disciplines but rather to evaluate scientific initiatives. Procedures should be developed that would permit scientific advisory committees and peer review panels to compare competing initiatives and reach unambiguous recommendations about priority, based on criteria such as scientific significance, breadth of interest, potential for new discoveries and understanding, possible contributions to the improvement of health, and the feasibility and logistics of the proposal. The committee believes that this should not be perceived as an attempt to empower government administrators to be central planners; rather, it is the committee's intent to establish a high-level priority-setting process with a wide range of input from all sponsors and performers of health research. Many issues were brought before the committee that were outside of the committee's charge. Many of these dealt with structural aspects of the Executive Branch that the committee was not able to address. These included: (1) the role of the research components of ADAMHA and their relationship to the research institutes in NIH, (2) the role of the Assistant Secretary for Health in oversight of research sponsored by NIH and ADAMHA, and (3) the role of federal laboratories in facilitating technology transfer. The committee believes that these items should be on the agenda of OSTP and a health FCCSET to encourage open debate.

The committee also deliberated extensively on the issue of 2-year congressional budget appropriations for the federal agencies that sponsor R&D. Whereas assessment of research needs would be conducted annually, including appropriate congressional testimony and progress reports from the various agencies, a rolling 2-year funding cycle could set minimum budget levels for particular institutes and programs. Under these circumstances, funding could be initiated at the beginning of each fiscal year without long delays, and this would lessen researcher anxiety about the priority level at which grants will be awarded. Such planning would also diminish the requirement that agencies arbitrarily reduce the level of previous awards because of unanticipated changes in funding levels. Although Congress would retain the option to reduce funding in the second year of a 2-year cycle, the actual history of overall budgetary stability suggests that such decreases would be unlikely. Congress is likely to avoid such midcycle changes in the interest of stability in the research environment. Although there are many positive aspects to a 2-year budget cycle for federal research agencies, the committee did not believe it was within its charge to recommend such a policy change.

Improving Communication and Cooperation Among Research Sponsors

Recommendation 6.3: The committee recommends that sponsors and researchers explore ways to share facilities and equipment among research institutions, industry, and government.

The committee also heard suggestions that institutions offset some of the high costs of research facilities and equipment by entering into cooperative regional agreements to share these expensive resources. Even if this cannot be done on a widespread basis, limited cooperation can further advances in health research and possibly can reduce unnecessary duplication of capital investments.

As equipment and facilities costs continue to soar, cooperative sharing should reduce the need to duplicate investment in physical infrastructure.

Understandably, there are difficulties with proprietary rights and maintaining intellectual freedoms. However, the model of cooperation employed by the National Institute of Standards and Technology sets a precedent for the success of these types of ventures. This could be achieved by employing the GUIRR structure proposed. All sponsors and performers of health research should explore ways to increase sharing of facilities and equipment. Even though conflict of interest must be avoided, the committee is convinced that cooperative agreements can arise without compromising the integrity of researchers or institutions.

Foundations and Voluntary Health Agencies

Recommendation 6.4: The committee recommends that foundations and voluntary health organizations maintain their support for new lines of investigation and research projects that, for political or structural reasons, NIH and ADAMHA cannot fund.

Traditionally, foundations and voluntary health agencies have been key supporters of interdisciplinary or innovative projects or of those projects that, for political or other reasons, are difficult to support with federal funds. Although nonprofit organizations will never have the resources to rival federal funding for health sciences research, they can respond to new lines of inquiry faster than the government bureaucracy allows. Furthermore, the disease-specific nature of voluntary health agencies provides them with a greater focus for supporting innovative ideas in specific areas of investigation as well as for funding trainees.

Although the committee believes that foundations and voluntary health agencies are integral to the health research enterprise, it emphasizes that these organizations must not be considered substitutes for federal support. Rather, these organizations should supplement federal efforts and fill in gaps in support in specific areas of research.

SCIENTIST RESPONSIBILITIES

Federal health research allocation policies often have emerged piecemeal out of the continuing political process. Policy decisions largely reflect scientific, political, and economic influences. The sponsors of health research need to work toward common goals with the research community in order to provide an optimum environment for health research. The committee's recommendations to now have focused primarily on the responsibilities of the sponsors. Little has been said about the role of research scientists and their responsibilities to the research system. Indeed, the key to a viable system is the active participation of scientists in all aspects of the research enterprise, including priority setting and allocation policy.

The committee concluded that research scientists could take actions that would help to improve the future success of the enterprise beyond their own commitment to specific research projects. Scientists should assume a more active role in the policy decision-making process and should champion the overall needs of the research establishment. Health research is a long-term investment, and scientists need to express their views to governmental representatives so that Congress and the Executive Branch can set national research priorities. Scientists also have a responsibility to serve on peer review panels; to review journal articles; and to provide advice on policy boards of the federal government, private foundations, and charitable organizations.

The committee believes that scientists should become more involved in improving the public's understanding of science. Negative publicity about science and scientists seems to be uppermost in the public consciousness in recent years. A very small number of highly publicized cases of alleged scientific misconduct and fraud are cited by some to be the tip of an iceberg of deception and misconduct pervading the scientific community. On the other hand, members of the scientific community have argued that the high degree of methodological reproducibility establishes the sound basis of scientific observation. Researchers must continue to show high regard for animal welfare and the proper handling of toxic wastes in order to avoid negative ramifications on the research establishment.

To improve the public's opinion of science, the committee believes that scientists must strive to rid the system of misconduct; they must cooperate fully with their institutions and research sponsors in cases of suspected wrongdoing. Also, scientists need to help prevent overreaction to these unfortunate incidents that could easily stigmatize the field. The committee endorses the recommendations of a recent IOM study group report, *The Responsible Conduct of Research in the Health Sciences*,[4] which includes recommendations that scientists, individually, as well as through professional societies and other organizations, promote high ethical standards in the conduct of research. Failing to address these concerns in the rapidly paced and highly competitive realm of modern biomedical research could have serious consequences, for each new case of scientific misconduct increases the possibility of federal regulation. The committee is concerned that legislatively mandated guidelines for ethical conduct and scientific reporting could impede research activities and increase research costs.

A CALL TO ACTION

Many of the problems, issues, and opportunities considered by this committee have been tackled before by the scientific community and by advisors to and within government. Despite numerous recommendations by those various groups, no decision to act has been made, and the basic problems therefore have persisted. The present analysis has sought to include all of the sources of health sciences research support in order to provide a more comprehensive overview of current trends for all components of the research establishment. The committee concluded that an imbalance in support among the components of the research enterprise needs to be addressed immediately to ensure a viable system into the next century. Effective and longer-term corrections will be made only when those who are examining the issues have the authority to act on their conclusions as well. Therefore, the committee believes that in order to begin resolving the problems discussed in this report and to make the best use of available research funds, ongoing communication among all research sponsors and the whole of the scientific community is vitally important. Only in this way can the wisdom invested in the enterprise be applied in a continuing effort of self-regulation and success.

REFERENCES

1. National Research Council. 1989. Biomedical and Behavioral Research Scientists: Their Training and Supply. Washington, D.C.: National Academy Press.
2. Institute of Medicine. 1988. Resources for Clinical Investigation. Washington, D.C.: National Academy Press.
3. National Academy of Sciences, National Academy of Engineering, and the Institute of Medicine. 1989. National Issues in Science and Technology: V. Federal Science and Technology Budget Priorities, New Perspectives and Procedures. Washington, D.C.: National Academy Press.
4. Institute of Medicine. 1988. The Responsible Conduct of Research in the Health Sciences. Washington, D.C.: National Academy Press.

Appendix A

Tables

The following tables were assembled from data collected from the National Institutes of Health, the Alcohol, Drug Abuse, and Mental Health Administration, and other federal agencies sponsoring health research. These tables supplement the data depicted in the figures and appearing in the text.

TABLE A-1 National Support for Health R&D by Source, 1977-1989 (dollars in millions)

Year	Total	Government				Industry	Private Nonprofit
		Total Government	NIH	Other Federal	State and Local		
1977	5,568	3,734	2,280	1,116	338	1,614	220
1978	6,262	4,226	2,581	1,230	415	1,800	220
1979	7,133	4,786	2,953	1,368	465	2,093	254
1980	7,935	5,203	3,182	1,541	480	2,459	274
1981	8,703	5,413	3,333	1,515	564	2,998	292
1982	9,483	5,605	3,433	1,415	634	3,561	318
1983	10,634	6,112	3,789	1,610	712	4,145	377
1984	12,014	6,880	4,257	1,830	793	4,643	491
1985	13,408	7,665	4,828	1,963	874	5,244	500
1986	14,801	7,922	5,005	1,890	1,026	6,166	714
1987	16,827	8,973	5,851	1,976	1,146	7,130	725
1988*	18,729	9,726	6,291	2,163	1,272	8,620	744
1989*	20,575	10,547	6,792	2,415	1,339	9,259	770

*Estimate

SOURCES: National Science Foundation. 1989. Science and Technology Resources: Funding and Personnel. Publication No. 89-300. Washington, D.C. U.S. Department of Health and Human Services; Public Health Service. 1989. NIH Data Book 1989. Publication No. 89-1261. Bethesda, Md.: National Institutes of Health.

TABLE A-2 NIH and ADAMHA Appropriations in Current and Constant 1988 Dollars, 1945-1991 (dollars in millions)

Year	NIH Current	NIH Constant	ADAMHA Current	ADAMHA Constant
1945	3	26	--**	--
1950	59	369	--	--
1955	81	439	--	--
1960	381	1,826	--	--
1965	958	4,063	--	--
1970	1,444	4,828	--	--
1975	2,109	5,146	--	--
1976	2,238	4,971	--	--
1977	2,544	5,350	886	1,863
1978	2,842	5,568	939	1,838
1979	3,190	5,772	1,025	1,854
1980	3,429	5,652	1,019	1,676
1981	3,569	5,328	923	1,377
1982	3,642	5,531	758	1,041
1983	4,024	5,207	808	1,045
1984	4,476	5,468	845	1,031
1985	5,145	5,950	919	1,062
1986	5,494	6,087	927	1,026
1987	6,181	6,505	1,317	1,386
1988	6,667	6,667	1,374	1,374
1989*	7,144	6,744	1,867	1,775
1990*	7,576	6,749	2,643	2,377
1991*	7,930	6,741	2,844	2,417

NOTE: Constant 1988 dollars are calculated using the Biomedical Research and Development Price Index (BRDPI). The BRDPI was developed by the department of Commerce's Bureau of Economic Analysis to measure the effects of price changes in the inputs to research supported by NIH (Holloway and Reed, 1989). The values for 1988-1990 are estimates based on OMB projections of the implicit price deflator for GNP and its historical Relationship with changes in the BRDPI.

*Estimates
**Data not available

SOURCES: U.S. Department of Health and Human Services; Public Health Service. 1989 NIH Almanac. Publication No. 89-5. Bethesda, Md. National Institutes of Health. U.S. Department of Health and Human Services; Public Health Service. 1989. ADAMHA Data Source Book 1988. Rockville, Md.: Alcohol, Drug Abuse, and Mental Health Administration.

TABLE A-3 Centers for Disease Control Research Funding in Current and Constant 1988 Dollars, 1984-1990 (dollars in thousands)

Year	Total CDC		NIOSH		Other CDC	
	Current	Constant	Current	Constant	Current	Constant
1984	46,292	56,587	17,725	21,667	28,567	34,897
1985	45,647	52,827	20,353	23,555	25,294	29,253
1986	52,203	57,877	21,999	24,390	30,204	33,466
1987	65,394	69,108	23,998	25,361	41,396	43,565
1988*	87,642	87,642	24,438	24,438	63,204	63,204
1989*	100,562	95,530	24,748	23,510	75,814	71,596
1990	104,978	94,470	25,871	23,281	79,107	71,188

NOTE: BRDPI deflator

*Estimates

SOURCE: CDC Public Affairs Office, Document 7293A.

TABLE A-4 Department of Veterans Affairs R&D Appropriations in Current and Constant 1988 Dollars, 1979-1989 (dollars in thousands)

Year	Total		Medical Research *	Rehabilitation Research	Health Services R&D
	Current	Constant			
1979	121,622	220,075	111,758	6,480	3,374
1980	125,847	207,446	115,388	7,306	3,153
1981	140,070	209,111	127,680	9,140	3,250
1982	136,711	187,909	126,698	7,185	2,828
1983	154,839	200,362	141,052	10,001	3,786
1984	163,706	199,983	147,697	10,897	5,112
1985	187,269	216,577	165,557	15,277	6,435
1986	178,926	198,250	157,123	15,345	6,458
1987	190,798	200,796	164,914	17,760	8,124
1988	187,902	187,902	159,208	20,534	8,160
1989	207,491	195,892	179,102	18,994	9,395

NOTE: BRDPI deflator

*Excludes all appropriated funding for dioxion epidemiology study FY 1981-1989 conducted for the VA by the Centers for Disease Control and funding in FY 1988 for a contract for Womens Epidemiology study.

SOURCE: Data provided by the Department of Veterans Affairs.

TABLE A-5   National Science Foundation Obligations in Current and Constant 1988 Dollars, 1977-1991 (dollars in millions)

Year	Current	Constant
1977	791.77	1,453.85
1978	857.25	1,471.16
1979	926.93	1,464.58
1980	975.13	1,416.31
1981	1,035.27	1,367.06
1982	999.14	1,229.71
1983	1,099.68	1,301.00
1984	1,306.87	1,485.59
1985	1,507.07	1,656.12
1986	1,493.16	1,594.08
1987	1,626.67	1,684.27
1988	1,717.00	1,717.00
1989[a]	1,885.90	1,779.63
1990[a]	2,083.60	1,854.40
1991[a,b]	2,383.60	2,001.70

NOTE: BRDPI deflator

[a]Appropriations.
[b]Estimate.

SOURCE: National Science Foundation. 1987. Report on Funding Trends and Balance of Acitivities: National Science Foundation 1951-1988. NSF 88-3. Washington, D.C.

TABLE A-6   Appropriations for the United States Army Medical Research and Development Command in Current and Constant 1988 Dollars, 1980-1989 (dollars in thousands)

Year	Current	Constant
1980	82,756	136,415
1981	89,892	134,200
1982	123,335	169,524
1983	163,104	211,057
1984	237,091	289,630
1985	266,291	307,966
1986	269,200	298,273
1987	302,586	262,480
1988	262,480	262,480
1989	252,291	238,816

NOTE: BRDPI deflator.

SOURCE: Data Provided by the U.S. Army Medical Research and Development Command.

TABLE A-7 NIH Appropriations in Current and Constant 1988 Dollars and NIH Appropriations in Constant 1988 Dollars Less AIDS Research, 1977-1991 (dollars in millions)

Year	Current	Constant	Constant Dollars Less AIDS Research
1977	2,544	5,350	** --
1978	2,842	5,568	--
1979	3,190	5,772	--
1980	3,429	5,652	--
1981	3,569	5,328	--
1982	3,642	5,531	5,527
1983	4,024	5,207	5,179
1984	4,476	5,468	5,414
1985	5,145	5,950	5,876
1986	5,494	6,087	5,937
1987	6,181	6,505	6,240
1988	6,667	6,667	6,199
1989*	7,144	6.744	6,177
1990*	7,576	6,740	6,080
1991*	7,930	6,740	6,050

NOTE: BRDPI deflator

*Estimates
**Data not available

SOURCE: National Institutes of Health, Division of Research Grants.

TABLE A-8 NIH Budget Obligations, 1977-1989 (dollars in thousands)

Year	Total	Extramural	Intramural	Operations
1977	2,581,988	2,018,103	247,952	315,933
1978	2,828,012	2,258,885	284,916	284,211
1979	3,184,641	2,592,827	345,432	246,382
1980	3,428,842	2,800,832	377,923	250,087
1981	3,572,506	2,897,444	413,427	261,635
1982	3,643,461	2,925,908	451,730	265,823
1983	4,013,135	3,227,751	498,210	287,174
1984	4,493,553	3,637,832	539,514	316,207
1985	5,121,557	4,224,397	571,595	325,565
1986	5,296,977	4,327,001	571,602	398,374
1987	6,175,038	5,126,267	665,311	383,460
1988*	6,610,430	5,475,499	715,039	419,892
1989*	6,610,430	5,475,499	715,039	419,892

*Estimate

SOURCE: U.S. Department of Health and Human Services; Public Health Service. 1989. NIH Data Book Publication No. 90-1261. Bethesda, Md.: National Institutes of Health.

TABLE A-9 ADAMHA Appropriations in Current and Constant 1988 Dollars, 1977-1991 (dollars in millions)

Year	Total Appropriations		Research Funds	
	Current	Constant	Current	Constant
1977	886.0	1,822.8	152.8	314.4
1978	938.8	1,798.3	161.3	309.0
1979	1,025.2	1,855.1	196.0	354.7
1980	1,017.8	1,677.8	211.7	349.0
1981	923.1	1,378.1	206.6	308.4
1982	757.5	1,041.2	208.2	309.5
1983	808.0	1,045.6	239.2	309.5
1984	844.8	1,032.0	271.2	331.3
1985	918.8	1,062.6	303.8	351.3
1986	926.5	1,026.6	329.0	364.5
1987	1,317.3	1,386.3	329.0	364.5
1988	1,373.7	1,373.7	554.8	554.8
1989	1,867.3	1,680.4	727.0	654.2
1990*	2,643.4	2,377.7	727.0	653.9
1991*	2,843.5	2,416.9	941.0	799.9

NOTE: BRDPI deflator

*Estimates

SOURCE: U.S. Department of Health and Human Services; Public Health Service. ADAMHA Data Source Book, FY 1988. ADAMHA Program Analysis Report No. 89-18. Rockville, Md.: Alcohol, Drug Abuse, and Mental Health Administration.

TABLE A-10 ADAMHA Budget Allocations, 1977-1989 (dollars in millions)

Year	Research	Training	Community Programs	Programs Support	Total
1977	152.8	103.8	567.5	61.9	886.0
1978	161.3	101.6	611.7	64.2	938.8
1979	196.0	107.6	654.0	67.6	1,025.2
1980	211.7	105.9	626.3	73.9	1,017.8
1981	206.6	94.4	543.4	78.7	923.1
1982	208.2	63.2	428.0	58.1	757.5
1983	239.2	37.9	468.0	62.9	808.0
1984	271.2	38.3	469.0	66.3	844.8
1985	303.8	43.0	503.0	69.0	918.8
1986	329.0	39.2	494.8	63.5	926.5
1987	411.3	38.6	800.3	67.1	1,317.3
1988	478.0	40.7	786.3	68.7	1,373.7
1989	542.5	39.8	902.3	78.1	1,562.7

SOURCE: U.S. Department of Health and Human Services; Public Health Service. ADAMHA Data Source Book, FY 1988. ADAMHA Program Analysis Report No. 89-18. Rockville, Md.: Alcohol, Drug Abuse, and Mental Health Administration.

TABLE A-11 NIH Competitive Grant Applications Submitted, Number Awarded and Approval, Award, and Success Rates, 1970-1991 (dollars in thousands)

Year	Requested		Awarded		Rates		
	Number	Amount	Number	Amount	Approval	Award	Success
1970	7,634	393,821	2,580	110,169	67.0	50.2	33.7
1971	7,579	430,476	2,691	132,960	68.8	50.8	35.1
1972	8,596	542,857	3,624	194,135	69.9	59.0	41.5
1973	9,306	668,609	2,591	166,010	71.3	38.9	27.7
1974	9,448	734,256	4,540	307,280	74.7	58.2	44.6
1975	10,093	812,373	4,663	298,328	74.4	60.6	45.3
1976	10,050	891,192	3,464	263,002	71.3	48.3	34.4
1977	13,304	261,825	3,839	306,834	74.0	38.7	28.7
1978	14,502	1,398,719	5,200	420,796	77.6	45.3	35.3
1979	14,458	1,525,662	5,937	525,126	77.5	51.6	40.2
1980	14,142	1,562,346	4,785	471,840	79.3	42.3	33.6
1981	15,731	1,899,883	5,107	545,270	82.3	39.2	32.3
1982	16,989	2,227,363	5,026	564,621	84.7	34.7	29.4
1983	16,798	2,305,448	5,388	643,424	85.9	37.2	32.0
1984	16,794	2,403,389	5,492	731,981	87.4	37.3	32.6
1985	18,673	2,954,883	6,245	918,102	89.2	37.3	33.3
1986	19,119	3,120,455	6,149	914,151	89.5	35.8	32.1
1987	18,470	3,319,726	6,446	1,119,634	90.7	38.3	34.8
1988	19,119	3,728,726**	6,212	1,098,537	91.6	35.3	32.3
1989	19,535	--	5,383	--	93.5	29.9	27.6
1990*	19,500	--	4,600	--	94.5	25.0	24.0
1991	19,500	--	5,100	--	94.5	25.1	24.0

*Estimates
**Data not available

SOURCE: National Institutes of Health, Division of Research Grants.

TABLE A-12   Allocation of NIH Extramural Awards by Activity, 1970-1988 (dollars in thousands)

Year	Total Amount Awarded	Research Projects	Centers/ Other Grants	R&D Contracts	NRSA Traning	Other
1970	881,426	438,283	187,265	99,828	151,654	4,397
1971	1,005,426	490,683	209,855	148,416	154,007	2,464
1972	1,253,650	589,066	237,419	221,537	158,863	46,765
1973	1,241,201	617,426	221,047	250,505	116,077	36,147
1974	1,680,663	788,647	312,159	357,970	187,399	34,487
1975	1,735,283	849,593	298,447	398,080	157,693	31,469
1976	1,830,492	909,063	366,763	410,886	123,092	20,688
1977	2,015,157	996,829	438,887	430,118	131,551	17,773
1978	2,252,138	1,146,845	491,153	451,598	148,528	14,013
1979	2,590,417	1,401,991	549,664	474,992	149,310	14,460
1980	2,788,598	1,594,665	566,400	432,374	182,750	12,409
1981	2,883,673	1,767,142	564,213	366,928	181,720	3,669
1982	2,930,054	1,834,432	573,286	358,709	156,332	7,295
1983	3,246,415	2,098,550	603,716	370,334	171,103	2,711
1984	3,657,638	2,404,846	682,121	394,708	173,239	2,725
1985	4,248,136	2,784,832	806,513	417,725	223,962	15,104
1986	4,426,607	2,928,820	810,327	462,564	217,149	7,747
1987	5,194,187	3,487,183	914,005	544,356	238,791	9,852
1988	5,544,828	3,764,791	962,529	565,094	245,661	6,753
TOTAL	51,405,990	30,893,687	9,795,769	7,156,722	3,268,882	290,930

SOURCE: National Institutes of Health, Division of Research Grants.

TABLE A-13 NIH Allocations for Research Project Grants, 1978-1990 (dollars in millions)

Year	Total RPGs		R01		P01		Other	
	Number	Amount	Number	Amount	Number	Amount	Number	Amount
1979	15,770	1,402.0	14,722	1,118.6	498	260.1	550	23.3
1980	16,683	1,594.7	15,463	1,267.9	535	297.5	685	29.2
1981	16,908	1,767.1	15,549	1,402.6	549	325.4	810	39.1
1982	16,334	1,834.4	14,826	1,456.4	557	327.2	951	50.9
1983	17,212	2,098.6	15,421	1,665.3	574	357.5	1,217	75.8
1984	17,761	2,404.8	15,757	1,907.5	571	393.2	1,433	104.1
1985	18,905	2,784.8	16,504	2,174.6	630	461.5	1,771	148.8
1986	19,201	2,928.8	16,403	2,213.4	638	485.6	2,160	229.8
1987	20,213	3,487.2	16,868	2,517.9	638	589.0	2,610	380.3
1988	20,867	3,764.8	16,871**	2,564.2	770	634.8	3,226	565.8
1989*	20,681	4,300.0	-	3,800.0	-	-	-	-
1990*	20,316	4,200.0	-	3,740.0	-	-	-	-

*Estimate
**Data not available

SOURCE: U.S. Department of Health and Human Services; Public Health Service. 1989. NIH Data Book Publication No. 90-1261. Bethesda, Md.: National Institutes of Health.

TABLE A-14   Average Size of NIH Research Project Grant Awards in Current and Constant 1988 Dollars, 1977-1991 (dollars in thousands)

Year	Current	Constant
1977	82.2	181.2
1978	88.1	166.7
1979	92.1	165.0
1980	97.8	161.2
1981	107.1	159.9
1982	114.6	157.5
1983	123.7	160.0
1984	138.0	168.6
1985	150.2	173.7
1986	154.6	171.3
1987	175.4	184.6
1988	186.8	186.8
1989	198.0	186.9
1990*	206.0	184.0
1991*	218.0	185.0

NOTE: BRDPI deflator

*Estimates

SOURCE: U.S. Department of Health and Human Services; Public Health Service. 1989. NIH Data Book Publication No. 90-1261. Bethesda, Md.: National Institutes of Health.

TABLE A-15   Average Award Length in Years of Competing Traditional Research Project (R01) Awards 1977-1989

Year	Average Length
1977	3.19
1978	3.14
1979	3.18
1980	3.33
1981	3.34
1982	3.33
1983	3.25
1984	3.26
1985	3.30
1986	3.50
1987	3.75
1988	3.92
1989*	4.00

*Estimate

SOURCE: U.S. Department of Health and Human Services; Public Health Service. 1989. NIH Data Book Publication No. 90-1261. Bethesda, Md.: National Institutes of Health.

TABLE A-16   NIH Support for Research Centers in Current and Constant 1988 Dollars, 1970-1988 (dollars in millions)

Year	Number		Amount	
	Total	GCRCs	Current	Constant
1970	301	93	93,88	306,041
1971	332	82	119,584	369,659
1972	376	83	142,756	420,359
1973	389	83	150,933	424,212
1974	420	89	167,625	442,865
1975	398	84	179,676	428,815
1976	536	87	233,295	518,218
1977	574	83	284,804	585,928
1978	597	82	314,016	601,497
1979	664	82	339,391	614,128
1980	539	76	335,302	552,712
1981	520	75	339,425	506,728
1982	521	75	347,562	477,724
1983	501	75	375,710	486,169
1984	529	75	430,974	526,478
1985	572	78	483,345	558,988
1986	580	78	482,454	534,559
1987	582	78	536,090	564,181
1988	621	78	573,578	573,578

NOTE: BRDPI deflator

SOURCE: U.S. Department of Health and Human Services; Public Health Service. 1989. NIH Data Book Publication No. 90-1261. Bethesda, Md.: National Institutes of Health.

TABLE A-17   NCI Support for Cancer Centers in Current and
Constant 1988 Dollars, 1972-1989 (dollars in thousands)

Year	Support		Number of Centers
	Current	Constant	
1972	10,090	30,373	40
1973	13,002	37,351	44
1974	17,575	47,474	52
1975	30,096	73,441	56
1976	47,803	108,545	64
1977	55,132	115,945	56
1978	60,348	118,190	67
1979	64,364	116,475	68
1980	67,421	111,146	64
1981	71,408	106,611	57
1982	74,996	103,087	56
1983	77,372	100,119	60
1984	79,211	96,764	59
1985	84,957	98,250	57
1986	88,426	97,968	59
1987	95,819	100,841	60
1988	100,427	100,427	59
1989	101,345	95,681	54
1990[*]	101,345	90,608	49

NOTE: BRDPI deflator

[*]Estimate

SOURCE: Institute of Medicine. 1989. A Stronger Cancer Centers
Program.   Washington, D.C.: National Academy Press.

TABLE A-18 Indirect Cost Proportion of Total Cost for NIH Research Grants, 1970-1988

Year	Total Cost	Indirect Cost	Ratio
1970	539,597,544	111,119,387	20.6
1971	617,801,494	131,741,697	21.3
1972	744,780,557	165,591,370	22.2
1973	790,791,110	180,149,574	22.8
1974	996,954,028	241,976,934	24.3
1975	1,070,859,608	266,204,944	24.9
1976	1,196,827,984	315,972,870	26.4
1977	1,351,011,225	358,952,309	26.6
1978	1,543,093,824	416,671,615	27.0
1979	1,844,373,212	512,324,316	27.8
1980	2,048,917,556	586,300,309	28.6
1981	2,222,779,742	654,281,299	29.4
1982	2,300,561,863	689,889,818	30.0
1983	2,584,500,903	791,537,709	30.6
1984	2,958,251,185	921,626,908	31.2
1985	3,412,862,947	1,069,491,642	31.3
1986	3,562,457,200	1,119,070,366	31.4
1987	4,188,140,948	1,311,234,378	31.3
1988	4,511,317,225	1,386,951,712	30.7
TOTAL	38,485,880,155	11,231,089,157	29.2

NOTE: Nominal dollars

SOURCE: National Institutes of Health, Division of Research Grants.

TABLE A-19 Number of NIH Full-Time-Equivalent Training Positions (FTTPs), 1977-1988

Year	Total	Predoctoral	Postdoctoral
1977	10,198	5,130	5,068
1978	11,123	5,540	5,583
1979	11,197	5,349	5,848
1980	10,664	5,095	5,569
1981	10,695	5,353	5,342
1982	10,406	5,081	5,325
1983	10,570	5,254	5,316
1984	10,514	5,149	5,365
1985	10,624	4,963	5,661
1986	10,382	5,011	5,371
1987	11,181	5,438	5,743
1988	11,329	5,560	5,769

SOURCE: U.S. Department of Health and Human Services; Public Health Service. 1989. NIH Data Book Publication No. 90-1261. Bethesda, Md.: National Institutes of Health.

TABLE A-20 ADAMHA Obligations for Research Training in Current and Constant 1988 Dollars and Number of Full-Time-Equivalent Training Positions (FTTPs), 1978-1988 (dollars in millions)

Year	Obligations		Number of FTTPs		
	Current	Constant	Predoctoral	Postdoctoral	Total
1978	16.923	33.163	1,178	531	1,709
1979	17.184	31.116	941	592	1,533
1980	19.963	32.929	789	604	1,393
1981	20.810	31.088	808	615	1,423
1982	17.167	23.612	652	594	1,246
1983	17.127	22.175	579	579	1,158
1984	17.157	20.973	585	546	1,131
1985	20.794	24.065	570	561	1,131
1986	19.818	21.972	547	518	1,065
1987	23.535	24.872	639	609	1,248
1988	23.758	23.758	694	573	1,267

NOTE: BRDPI deflator. Data for 1987-1988 are non-AIDS.

SOURCE: Alcohol, Drug Abuse and Mental Health Administration. 1989. ADAMHA NRSA Research Training Tables, FY 1988. Program Analysis Report No. 89-15. Washington, D.C.: U.S. Department of Health and Human Services.

TABLE A-21 Number of Appointments in NIH Research Training Programs by Academic Level, 1980-1988

Year	M.D.	Ph.D.	Predoctoral	Total
1980	2,092	3,656	6,343	12,091
1981	2,051	3,449	6,682	12,182
1982	2,094	3,302	6,533	11,929
1983	2,224	3,260	6,648	12,132
1984	2,296	3,117	6,589	12,002
1985	2,429	3,304	6,356	12,089
1986	2,432	3,103	6,083	11,618
1987	2,454	3,065	6,237	11,756
1988	2,569	3,071	6,188	11,828

SOURCE: U.S. Department of Health and Human Services. 1989. NIH Data Book 1989. National Institutes of Health Publication No. 90-1261. Bethesda, Md.

TABLE A-22 Re-Allocation of the NIH Extramural Budget Under No Real Growth Scenario, 1988-2000 (dollars in thousands)

Function/Mechanism	1988	1989	1990	1995	2000
Obligations	6,740,874	6,774,059	6,774,059	6,774,059	6,621,643
Institutes/Research Divisions	9,461,980	6,589,204	6,621,643	6,621,643	6,621,643
Extramural Budget	5,475,494	5,583,033	5,610,518	5,610,518	5,610,518
Intramural Budget	714,701	728,766	732,354	732,354	732,354
Program Management	271,403	276,747	278,109	278,109	278,109
National Library of Medicine	67,426	68,757	69,095	69,095	69,095
Office of the Director	61,477	62,690	62,999	62,999	62,999
Building and Facilities	19,170	19,549	19,645	19,645	19,645
Project Grants	3,764,950	3,827,727	3,822,446	3,724,262	3,640,104
Centers/Other Grants	962,592	987,080	997,550	1,025,603	1,053,655
Contracts	497,175	506,939	509,435	509,435	509,435
NRSA Training	238,732	254,586	267,061	323,166	379,271
Construction	0	6,700	14,026	28,053	28,053
Totals	5,463,448	5,583,033	5,610,518	5,610,518	5,610,518

TABLE A-23 Re-Allocation of the NIH Extramural Budget Under Two Percent Real Growth Scenario, 1988-2000 (dollars in thousands)

Function/Mechanism	1988	1989	1990	1995	2000
Obligations	6,610,430	6,740,874	6,774,059	7,479,109	8,257,540
Institutes/Research Divisions	6,461,890	6,589,204	6,621,643	7,310,829	8,071,746
Extramural Budget	5,475,494	5,583,033	5,610,518	6,194,465	6,839,190
Intramural Budget	714,701	728,766	732,354	808,578	892,735
Program Management	271,403	276,747	278,109	307,055	339,013
National Library of Medicine	67,426	68,757	69,095	76,287	84,227
Office of the Director	61,477	62,690	62,999	69,556	76,795
Building and Facilities	19,170	19,549	19,645	21,689	23,947
Project Grants	3,764,950	3,827,727	3,822,446	4,111,886	4,437,267
Centers/Other Grants	962,592	987,080	997,550	1,132,348	1,284,400
Contracts	497,175	506,939	509,435	562,457	620,998
NRSA Training	238,732	254,586	267,061	356,801	462,329
Construction	0	6,700	14,026	30,972	34,196
Totals	5,463,448	5,583,033	5,610,518	6,194,465	6,839,190

TABLE A-24 Re-Allocation of the NIH Extramural Budget Under Four Percent Real Growth Scenario, 1988-2000 (dollars in thousands)

Function/Mechanism	1988	1989	1990	1995	2000
Obligations	6,610,430	6,740,874	6,774,059	8,241,679	10,027,262
Institutes/Research Divisions	6,461,890	6,589,204	6,621,643	8,056,241	9,801,649
Extramural Budget	5,475,494	5,583,033	5,610,518	6,826,053	8,304,937
Intramural Budget	714,701	728,766	732,354	891,020	1,084,062
Program Management	271,403	276,747	278,109	338,362	411,669
National Library of Medicine	67,426	68,757	69,095	84,065	102,278
Office of the Director	61,477	62,690	62,999	76,648	93,254
Building and Facilities	19,170	19,549	19,645	23,901	29,079
Project Grants	3,764,950	3,830,519	3,828,056	4,555,025	5,438,073
Centers/Other Grants	962,592	987,080	997,550	1,247,802	1,559,667
Contracts	497,175	506,939	509,435	619,806	754,088
NRSA Training	238,732	251,795	261,450	369,289	511,584
Construction	0	6,700	14,026	34,130	41,525
Totals	5,463,448	5,583,033	5,610,518	6,826,053	8,304,937

Appendix B

Biographies of Committee Members

FLOYD E. BLOOM, M.D. *(Chair)*, Chairman, Department of Neuropharmacology, Research Institute of Scripps Clinic, La Jolla, California. Trained as a neuropharmacologist after developing an interest in the sites and mechanisms by which drugs control hypertension within the brain, Dr. Bloom worked at the National Institute of Mental Health, and at Yale University before moving to the Salk Institute in 1975. After a productive period of research there, he transferred his base of operations to the nearby Research Institute of Scripps Clinic in 1983 to re-establish the medical environment which has always played a major shaping role in his selection of research topics. An active neuroscientist and past Chairman of the National Academy's neurobiology section, Dr. Bloom has pursued science policy issues through his election as president of the Society of Neuroscience, and through election to the Council of the IOM and the Board of Directors for the American Association for the Advancement of Science. He previously has served the Academy Complex as the study director for the Third Five Year Outlook on Science and Technology, and as chairman of the COSEPUP Briefing Paper for OSTP on the Neurosciences.

HENRY J. AARON, Ph.D., Senior Fellow, The Brookings Institution, Washington, D.C. Dr. Aaron joined the staff of the Brookings Institution as a senior fellow in 1968. He became a member of the Department of Economics at the University of Maryland in 1967 and was promoted to professor in 1973. He is a member of the Board of Directors of Abt Associates, Inc. He attended college at UCLA and graduate school at

Harvard University, from which he received a Ph.D. in economics. Before joining the faculty at Maryland and the staff at Brookings, he served as a staff member of the President's Council of Economic Advisers. His tenure at Brookings and the University of Maryland was interrupted in 1977 and 1978 when he served as assistant secretary for planning and evaluation at the Department of Health, Education and Welfare. He chaired the 1979 Advisory Council on Social Security and chaired the panel on housing allowance experiments of the Department of Housing and Urban Development. He has been a distinguished policy fellow at the University of California's Graduate School of Public Policy and a visiting professor at Harvard University. He is a member of the Institute of Medicine.

JACK D. BARCHAS, M.D., Associate Dean for Neuroscience at UCLA School of Medicine and Professor in the Department of Psychiatry and Biobehavioral Sciences. Dr. Barchas obtained his medical degree at Yale, and took his internship at the Pritzker School of Medicine of the University of Chicago. He received his postdoctoral training at the NIH, and his psychiatry residency at Stanford where he was a faculty member through 1989. At Stanford, he held the Nancy Friend Pritzker Professorship and was Associate Chairman of the Department of Psychiatry and Behavioral Sciences. Dr. Barchas is a member of the Institute of Medicine and chairs the Board on Biobehavioral Science and Mental Disorders. The thrust of Dr. Barchas' research has dealt with neuroregulators and behavior. A major theme of his efforts has been devoted to: (1) identification of previously unrecognized neuroregulators, especially neuropeptides; (2) study of fundamental control mechanisms for the neuroregulators, using analytical neurochemistry and biochemical neuroanatomy; and (3) exploration of the roles of neuroregulators in animal and human behavior as well as in human mental disorders and addictive states.

RONALD BRESLOW, Ph.D., Mitchell Professor of Chemistry, Department of Chemistry, Columbia University, New York, New York. Dr. Breslow is a physical organic chemist who also works on biochemical problems. He and his students and postdoctoral fellows design new molecules, synthesize them, and then determine if their properties are as interesting as was hoped. An important example is the cyclopropenyl cation, the simplest aromatic system. In another area he designed and studied catalysts that were the first to be described as artificial enzymes, and he created and named the field of biochemetic chemistry. Dr. Breslow has been a faculty member of the Columbia chemistry department since 1956, but he has also served on the Board of Trustees of Rockefeller University and is a past chairman of the chemistry section of the National Academy of Sciences.

HOWARD E. FREEMAN, Ph.D., Professor of Sociology, University of California at Los Angeles. Professor Freeman joined UCLA in 1974 after serving as the Ford Foundation's social science advisor for Mexico, Central America, and the Caribbean. Dr. Freeman was the founding director of UCLA's Institute for Social Science Research, a position he held from 1974 until 1981. During his directorship, ISSR became a national policy research and evaluation center, undertaking applied studies in a broad range of social problem areas. He served as chair of his department from 1985 to 1989. Prior appointments include Brandeis University, where he was Morse Professor of Urban Studies, Harvard University, and Russell Sage Foundation. Dr. Freeman has published extensively in the health and mental health fields, on the post-hospital experience of mental patients, on policy issues in the delivery of health services, and on applied research methods. His monograph, *The Mental Patient Comes Home*, was awarded the Hofheimer Prize of the American Psychiatric Association. He is the co-editor of the *Handbook of Medical Sociology*, now in its fourth edition. Professor Freeman's text with Peter H. Rossi, *Evaluation: A Systematic Approach*, also in its fourth edition, is used widely in social program evaluation courses each year. He is the co-editor of *Evaluation Review*, and on the editorial boards of other social research and health care journals. He serves as a consultant to national foundations, a number of government groups, and several international research organizations.

HANNA HOLBORN GRAY, Ph.D., President and Professor of History, The University of Chicago, Chicago, Illinois. Dr. Gray became the 10th President of the University of Chicago on July 1, 1978, after having served as provost and acting president at Yale University. She is an historian with special interests in the history of humanism, political and historical thought and politics in the Renaissance and Reformation. She taught at Bryn Mawr from 1953 to 1954, Harvard from 1955 to 1960, and the University o Chicago from 1961 to 1974. She is a fellow of the American Academy of Arts and Sciences; a member of the Renaissance Society of America the American Philosophical Society, the National Academy of Education and the Board of Overseers of Harvard University; and a trustee of Bryn Mawr College, the National Humanities Center, the Andrew W. Mello Foundation, the Howard Hughes Medical Institute, and the Center fo Advanced Study in the Behavioral Sciences. In addition, Dr. Gray is member of the boards of directors of J.P. Morgan & Company/Morga Guarantee, the Cummins Engine Company, Atlantic Richfield Compan and Ameritech. Dr. Gray received her B.A. from Bryn Mawr College an her Ph.D. in history from Harvard. She also holds honorary degrees fro a number of institutions of higher learning.

BERNADINE HEALY, M.D., Chairman, Research Institute of The Cleveland Clinic Foundation, Cleveland, Ohio. Dr. Healy graduated from Vassar College (1965) and Harvard Medical School (1970) and was a professor of medicine and cardiology at the Johns Hopkins University School of Medicine through the mid-1980s. During 1984-85, she was deputy science advisor and associate director of the Office of Science and Technology Policy. Dr. Healy is currently vice-chairman of the President's Council of Advisors on Science and Technology (President Bush's advisory panel under Dr. Allan Bromley) and serves on the Special Medical Advisory Committee of the Department of Veterans Affairs. Besides being a member of the Institute of Medicine, she is chairman of the Office of Technology Assessment's Advisory Panel for New Developments in Biotechnology and serves on the Director's Advisory Committee/National Institutes of Health and on the Council on Research and Development of the Ohio Board of Regents. She was president of the American Heart Association (1988-89) and the American Federation for Clinical Research (1983-84), and presently serves on the Board of Overseers of Harvard College and several corporate boards.

SAMUEL HELLMAN, M.D., Dean, Division of Biological Sciences and the Pritzker School of Medicine, and Vice President for the Medical Center, University of Chicago, Chicago, Illinois. Dr. Hellman assumed his duties at the University of Chicago in September 1988. Prior to this, he was physician-in-chief of the Memorial Sloan-Kettering Hospital for Cancer and Allied Diseases from 1983-1988 and concurrently held the Benno C. Schmidt Chair in Clinical Oncology at Memorial Sloan-Kettering Cancer Center. In addition, Dr. Hellman was professor of radiation oncology at Cornell University Medical College from 1984-1988. Before joining Sloan-Kettering, Dr. Hellman served as chairman of the Department of Radiation Therapy at the Harvard Medical School where he was the Alvin T. and Viola D. Fuller-American Cancer Society Professor. He was director of the Joint Center for Radiation Therapy at the Harvard Medical School. Simultaneously, he served as chief of radiation therapy at a number of major hospitals in Boston. Dr. Hellman has been active in both clinical and laboratory investigation. He has been involved in studies of breast cancer and lymphoma. Dr. Hellman serves as chairman of the board of Allegheny College, where he received his B.S. degree magna cum laude in 1955. He is also a member of the Institute of Medicine. Dr. Hellman received the Richard and Hilda Rosenthal Foundation Award for Clinical Research of the American Association for Cancer Research in 1980.

MAUREEN HENDERSON, M.D., Professor of Epidemiology and Medicine, University of Washington, Fred Hutchinson Cancer Research Center, Seattle, Washington. Dr. Henderson began her career in preventive medicine and clinical epidemiological research in London at St. Bartholomew's Hospital and extended it at the University of Maryland and Johns Hopkins University in Baltimore. She returned to research in Seattle after ten years in academic administration. She has maintained an active interest in preventive intervention trials and is currently head of the Cancer Prevention Research Program at the Fred Hutchinson Cancer Research Center. Her initial research was in the prevention of chronic lung disease. She then became a founding investigator in the multicenter national trials to control hypertension and prevent coronary heart disease. Most recently, she has been responsible for one of the ground breaking research programs in cancer prevention. Dr. Henderson obtained her medical and public health degrees from the University of Durham in England.

RALPH HORWITZ, M.D., Professor of Medicine and Epidemiology at the Yale University School of Medicine, New Haven, Connecticut. Dr. Horwitz is co-director of the Robert Wood Johnson Clinical Scholars Program and chief of the General Medicine Section. In his research, Dr. Horwitz has studied the fundamental methods used to evaluate the strategies of clinical care. He has conducted numerous investigations of the etiology, prognosis, and treatment of disease. Dr. Horwitz has proposed new methods for improving scientific design in non-experimental research and scientific quality in basic data, and he has demonstrated the pragmatic application and effectiveness of these methods. He was a recipient of the Henry J. Kaiser Family Foundation Faculty Scholar Award and the Alumni Fellow Award of the Pennsylvania State University. Dr. Horwitz is a member of the American Society for Clinical Investigation and the American Epidemiological Society. He is a fellow of the American College of Physicians and the American College of Epidemiology.

ERNEST G. JAWORSKI, Ph.D., Distinguished Science Fellow and Director of Biological Sciences, Corporate Research and Development, Monsanto Company, St. Louis, Missouri. Dr. Jaworski has been with Monsanto since 1952 and currently actively oversees a large group of scientists whose research is devoted to several areas: plant molecular biology, chemistry, molecular genetics, and mammalian cell biology. Dr. Jaworski's work has included research on fungicides, herbicides, residue metabolism, animal growth and nutrition, plant molecular and cellular biology, and human health care product discovery. He received both his M.S. degree and Ph.D. from Oregon State University in biochemistry. Some of his current professional activities include: board member of the NutraSweet Company; fellow, American Society for Advancement of Science; member, National

Research Council; member, UCLA Symposia Board; and board member of Oxford Glycosystems, Ltd.

GERALD L. KLERMAN, Ph.D., Professor of Psychiatry and Associate Chairman for Research, Department of Psychiatry, Cornell University Medical College, New York, New York. Dr. Klerman is a psychiatrist with major involvement in clinical research, particularly in the evaluation of treatments as they influence mental health policy. He received his B.A. from Cornell University in 1950, and his M.D. from New York University in 1954. Following internship and residency in internal medicine and neurology at Bellevue Hospital in New York (1954-1956), he took his psychiatric residency training in Boston at the Massachusetts Mental Health Center (1956-1958). He has served on the faculties of Harvard and Yale. From 1977-1980, he was the administrator of the Alcohol, Drug Abuse and Mental Health Administration in the Public Health Service for which he received a Superior Service Award from the Public Health Service. His research activities focus on securing a more firm scientific base for clinical psychiatry. For these activities he has won a number of awards, including the American Psychiatric Association Hofheimer Award, 1970; the Foundation Fund Award; the Anna Monika Prize; and the William Menninger Memorial Award from the American College of Physicians.

THOMAS LANGFITT, M.D. (ex officio member), President and Chief Executive Officer, The Glenmede Trust Company and the Pew Charitable Trusts, Philadelphia, Pennsylvania. Prior to joining Glenmede, Dr. Langfitt had been a faculty member at the University of Pennsylvania for twenty-five years. During that time he served as professor and director of the Division of Neurosurgery and was also vice president for health affairs. Over the course of his career he made numerous contributions toward the advancement of neurosurgery and neurosciences through research, teaching, professional affiliations, and more than 200 published articles. He is a graduate of Princeton University and the Johns Hopkins University School of Medicine. His post-graduate training in general surgery, neurosurgery, and research in the neurosciences was conducted at the Johns Hopkins Medical School and Hospital. Dr. Langfitt is a charter trustee of Princeton University. He serves on the boards of directors of the Sun Company and the New York Life Insurance Company and on the U.S. Board of SmithKline Beecham. He is a member of the Institute of Medicine and the American Philosophical Society, and serves on the Medical Advisory Committee of the General Motors Corporation.

JOSHUA LEDERBERG, Ph.D., University Professor, the Rockefeller University, New York, New York. Dr. Lederberg is a research geneticist and was educated at Columbia and Yale University, where he pioneered in the field of bacterial genetics with the discovery of genetic recombination in bacteria. In 1958, at the age of 33, Dr. Lederberg received the Nobel Prize in Physiology and Medicine for his work and subsequent research on bacterial agents. Dr. Lederberg was a professor of genetics at the University of Wisconsin and then at Stanford University School of Medicine, until he came to the Rockefeller University in 1978. At Stanford, he was also a professor of computer science, working in research in artificial intelligence in biochemistry and medicine. A member of the National Academy of Sciences since 1957, and a charter member of the Institute of Medicine, Dr. Lederberg has been active on many government advisory committees and boards, such as NIH study sections and the National Advisory Mental Health Council, and has served as chairman of the President's Cancer Panel. Dr. Lederberg played an active role in NASA's Mariner and Viking missions to Mars. He is also involved in national security affairs as a member of the Defense Science Board, and currently serves on the congressional Technology Assessment Advisory Council. He chairs Annual Reviews, Inc. a cooperative non-profit scientific publisher, and serves on the boards of the Chemical Industry Institute for Toxicology, and several foundations as well as the Procter and Gamble Co. and the Institute for Scientific Information. He is currently co-chair of the Carnegie Commission on Science, Technology and Government. Dr. Lederberg has been awarded numerous honorary D.Sc. and M.D. degrees as well as foreign membership in the Royal Society, London.

ARIEL G. LOEWY, Ph.D., Jack and Barbara Bush Professor in the Natural Sciences and Chairman, Department of Biology, Haverford College, Haverford, Pennsylvania. Dr. Loewy came to Haverford College in 1953 and was appointed chairperson of the department in 1954. He developed a new curriculum centered on molecular and cell biology and on undergraduate research. In his research, Dr. Loewy demonstrated that actin and myosin were present in non-muscle cells, purified Factor XIII from blood plasma and showed that it crosslinked fibrin with isopeptide bonds and discovered a cytomatrix of covalently-crosslinked superfine filaments. His recent work is concerned with an enzyme capable of depolymerizing crosslinked fibrin by breaking isopeptide bonds. For his work on Factor XIII, Dr. Loewy received in 1973 the James F. Mitchell Foundation International Award for Cardiovascular Research. Dr. Loewy received his B.S. and M.S. degrees from McGill University and his Ph.D. from the University of Pennsylvania. He received an NIH postdoctoral fellowship to work at the Department of Physical Chemistry at Harvard Medical School and a National Research Council Fellowship to work at the Biochemistry Department of Cambridge University in England.

DON K. PRICE, Ph.D., Professor of Public Management, Emeritus, John F. Kennedy School of Government, Harvard University, Cambridge, Massachusetts. Mr. Price wrote the classic science policy texts *The Scientific Estate* (1956), *Government and Science* (1954), and *America's Unwritten Constitution: Science, Religion, and Political Responsibility* (1983). His scholarship in other fields has been prolific as well, and he served for nearly twenty years as dean of the John F. Kennedy School of Government at Harvard University. As a science policymaker and advisor, he has served as deputy chairman of the Defense Department Research and Development Board, director of the Social Science Research Council, vice president of the Ford Foundation, board chairman of the Twentieth Century Fund, and president of the American Association for the Advancement of Science. He also worked with former President Herbert Hoover on the Hoover Commission study of the organization of the U.S. Presidency and served as consultant to the Executive Office of the President during three administrations. Mr. Price was educated at Vanderbilt and Oxford Universities, the latter during his tenure as a Rhodes scholar. Currently, he is Albert J. Weatherhead III and Richard W. Weatherhead Professor of Public Management, Emeritus in the John F. Kennedy School of Government at Harvard University.

KENNETH SHINE, M.D., Dean, School of Medicine, University of California at Los Angeles, Los Angeles, California. Prior to being named dean in 1986 Dr. Shine was professor and executive chair of the UCLA Department of Medicine. Dr. Shine is a noted heart researcher, cardiologist, and teacher with a special interest in ischemic heart disease. He is a past president of the American Heart Association. Dr. Shine was born in Worcester, Massachusetts, in 1935. He earned his bachelor's degree in biochemical sciences in 1957 and his doctor of medicine degree in 1961, both from Harvard. He served his internship and residency in medicine at Massachusetts General Hospital in Boston before coming to UCLA in 1969 as a National Institutes of Health Special Postdoctoral Fellow. From 1970 to 1971, he served as assistant professor of medicine at Harvard and director of cardiovascular training for Beth Israel Hospital in Boston. Dr. Shine returned to UCLA in 1971 as an assistant professor of medicine and director of the coronary care unit at the UCLA Medical Center. He was appointed associate professor in 1973, chief of the division of cardiology in 1975, professor in 1977, vice-chair of the Department of Medicine in 1979, and executive chair of the department in 1981. He has received the UCLA Department of Medicine's Teacher of the Year award three times and has authored over 50 research articles. He has been selected as a visiting professor to medical schools throughout the world.

238

P. DENNIS SMITH, Ph.D., Chairman, Department of Biological Sciences, Wayne State University, Detroit, Michigan. Dr. Smith received his undergraduate education in biology at Loyola College in Baltimore and his doctoral training in genetics at the University of North Carolina. Following a postdoctorate at the University of Connecticut, he joined the faculty of Emory University in Atlanta. At Emory, Dr. Smith organized the Interdepartmental Program in Genetics, serving as its first director from 1977 through 1983. In 1984, Dr. Smith accepted the position of professor and chairman of the Department of Biological Sciences at Southern Methodist University and, in 1989, joined Wayne State University in Detroit as professor and chairman of Biological Sciences. Dr. Smith's research program is focused on the analysis of DNA repair and mutagenesis in eukaryotes, using mutagen-sensitive strains of *Drosophila melanogaster*. He has received support from the National Institutes of Health, the Environmental Protection Agency, the Air Force, the American Cancer Society, and a variety of private research foundations.

Appendix C

Task Forces

Committee Members

FLOYD E. BLOOM (*Chair*), Chairman, Department of
Neuropharmacology, Research Institute of Scripps Clinic, La Jolla,
California
HENRY J. AARON, Senior Fellow, The Brookings Institution,
Washington, D.C.
MAUREEN M. HENDERSON, Professor of Epidemiology and
Medicine, University of Washington, Fred Hutchinson Cancer
Research Center, Seattle, Washington
DON K. PRICE, Professor of Public Management, Emeritus, John F.
Kennedy School of Government, Harvard University, Cambridge,
Massachusetts
HOWARD E. FREEMAN, Professor, Department of Sociology,
University of California at Los Angeles, Los Angeles, California

Invited Guests

ROBERT W. BERLINER, Professor of Physiology and Medicine, Emeritus, Department of Physiology, Yale University School of Medicine, New Haven, Connecticut

JOEL W. GOLDSTEIN, Deputy Associate Administrator for Extramural Programs & Director, Division of Program Analysis, Alcohol, Drug Abuse and Mental Health Administration, Rockville, Maryland

WILLIAM F. RAUB, Deputy Director, National Institutes of Health

PETER GREENWALD, Director, Division of Cancer Prevention and Control, National Cancer Institute, Bethesda, Maryland

TASK FORCE 2 - GOALS OF BIOMEDICAL RESEARCH

Committee Members

RALPH I. HORWITZ (*Chair*), Professor, Department of Medicine, Yale University, New Haven, Connecticut

HANNA H. GRAY, President and Professor of History, University of Chicago, Chicago, Illinois

ERNEST G. JAWORSKI, Distinguished Science Fellow and Director of Biological Sciences, Monsanto Company, St. Louis, Missouri

THOMAS W. LANGFITT, (ex officio member) President and Chief Executive Officer, The Glenmede Trust Company and the Pew Charitable Trusts, Philadelphia, Pennsylvania

Invited Guest

JUDITH RODIN, Phillip R. Allen Professor of Psychology, Professor of Medicine and Psychiatry, Yale University

TASK FORCE 3 - OPTIMIZING THE ENVIRONMENT FOR BIOMEDICAL RESEARCH

Committee Members

KENNETH I. SHINE (*Chair*), Dean, School of Medicine, University of California at Los Angeles, Los Angeles, California

SAMUEL HELLMAN, Dean, Division of Biological Sciences and the Pritzker School of Medicine, and Vice President for the Medical Center, University of Chicago, Chicago, Illinois

ARIEL G. LOEWY, Jack and Barbara Bush Professor in the Natural Sciences and Chairman, Department of Biology, Haverford College, Haverford, Pennsylvania

P. DENNIS SMITH, Chairman, Department of Biological Sciences, Wayne State University, Detroit, Michigan

JACK D. BARCHAS, Associate Dean for Neuroscience and Professor of Neuroscience and Biobehavioral Sciences, School of Medicine, University of California at Los Angeles, Los Angeles, California

Invited Guests

IVAN L. BENNETT, Professor of Medicine, New York University Medical Center, New York, New York

TONY MERRITT, Office of Grants and Contracts, University of Pennsylvania, Philadelphia, Pennsylvania

Appendix D

Respondents to Input Request

The following individuals responded to a request from the chairman to provide a position statement from themselves or for their respective organization on the allocation of health research resources. The affiliation noted in the following list reflects their official capacity at the time of the response.

DAVID BALTIMORE, Director, Whitehead Institute

MAURICE Q. BECTEL, President, Pharmaceutical Manufacturers Association Foundation, Inc.

ROSEMARY H. BRUNER, Administrative Director, The Hoffman-La Roche Foundation

PEDRO CUATRECASAS, Senior Vice President of Research and Development, Glaxo Research Laboratories, Glaxo, Inc.

JEAN FITZGERALD DUBOIS, Program Officer, W.M. Keck Foundation

L.A. FISK, Associate Administrator for Space Science and Applications, National Aeronautics and Space Administration

TIMOTHY S. GEE, Attending Physician, Hematology/Lymphoma Service, Memorial Sloan-Kettering Cancer Center

RICHARD J. GLASSOCK, President, National Kidney Foundation, Inc.

BERNADINE HEALY, President, American Heart Association

ROBERT W. KRAUSS, Executive Director, Federation of American Societies for Experimental Biology

RONALD KUNTZMAN, Vice President of Research and Development, Hoffman-La Roche, Inc.

KATHERINE McCARTER, President, Coalition for Health Funding
LYNN MORRISON, Director for Public Policy, American Federation for
Clinical Research
GERALD J. MOSSINGHOFF, President, Pharmaceutical Manufacturers
Association
JOHN PRATT, President, Association of Independent Research Institutes
at Whitehead Institute
RICHARD S. ROSS, Vice President for Medicine, Dean of the Medical
Faculty, The Johns Hopkins University School of Medicine
EDWARD M. SCOLNICK, President of Research, Merck Sharp &
Dohme Research Laboratories, Division of Merck & Co., Inc.
RICHARD S. SHARPE, Program Director, The John A. Hartford
Foundation, Inc.
SOLOMON H. SNYDER, Distinguished Service Professor of
Neuroscience, Pharmacology and Psychiatry, Department of
Neuroscience, The Johns Hopkins University
EDWIN C. WHITEHEAD, Whitehead Associates
DANIEL H. WINSHIP, Associate Deputy Chief Medical Director,
Department of Medicine and Surgery, Veterans Administration

Index